Pressure Area Care

D0315080

EDITED BY

Karen Ousey
RGN, ONC, PGDE, DPPN, BA, MA
Lecturer in Nursing
University of Salford
Salford
UK

Blackwell
Publishing

© 2005 by Blackwell Publishing Ltd

Editorial offices:
Blackwell Publishing Ltd, 9600 Garsington Road, Oxford OX4 2DQ, UK
    Tel: +44 (0)1865 776868
Blackwell Publishing Inc., 350 Main Street, Malden, MA 02148-5020, USA
    Tel: +1 781 388 8250
Blackwell Publishing Asia Pty Ltd, 550 Swanston Street, Carlton, Victoria 3053,
Australia
    Tel: +61 (0)3 8359 1011

First published 2005 by Blackwell Publishing Ltd

Library of Congress Cataloging-in-Publication Data

Pressure area care / edited by Karen Ousey. – 1st ed.
        p.   ;   cm.
     Includes bibliographical references and index.
     ISBN 1-4051-1225-5 (pbk. : alk. paper)
    1. Bedsores – Prevention.   2. Nursing.
     [DNLM: 1. Ducubitus Ulcer – nursing. WY 154.5 P935 2005]   I. Ousey,
Karen.
RL675.P686 2005
616.5'4505 – dc22

                                                        2004021824

ISBN-10 1-4051-1225-5
ISBN-13 978-14051-1225-3

A catalogue record for this title is available from the British Library

Set in 9/12 Palatino
by SNP Best-set Typesetter Ltd., Hong Kong
Printed and bound in India
by Replika Press Pvt. Ltd, Kundli

For further information on Blackwell Publishing, visit our website:
www.blackwellnursing.com

Contents

Foreword

The impetus to improve the care of patients at risk of, or with, pressure damage is growing. The formation, in 1997, of the European Pressure Ulcer Advisory Panel has led to the coordination of several multidisciplinary initiatives across Europe, including a pan-European prevalence study which demonstrated that over a fifth of hospital inpatients have pressure ulcers (23%). In an attempt to reduce the frequency of occurrence of pressure damage, guidelines have been produced and disseminated in many European languages. This drive to reduce the frequency of pressure damage is the very core of the EPUAP, with one of the main aims being: 'to improve the outcome for patients at risk of pressure damage'. But is this happening?

Few people acknowledge that pressure ulcers can be a primary cause of death. The recent death of 'Superman' himself, the actor Christopher Reeves, can, if the publicity statement is read carefully, be seen to be due to a pressure ulcer from which he developed septicaemia. He was an intelligent, articulate man with immense financial resources and constant daily care from a loving family as well as a team of round the clock carers, yet he still developed a pressure ulcer. How can this still happen in a world of technological advancements that allow us to deliver babies at 24 weeks gestation and to keep people with the most complex disease processes alive?

Pressure ulcers affect so many people across the world, yet their existence is widely unknown by the general public and ignored in the political arena. They are a fundamental aspect of nursing care, yet little time is devoted to their study in either pre- or post-registration training of nurses. Many trusts employ Nurse Specialists or even Nurse Consultants in tissue viability but their daily impact is restricted and they cannot be everywhere at once. Pressure area care is the responsibility of every single nurse and, whilst having a lead clinician focuses the mind and organises initiatives, from a strategic point of view it is the nurse at the bedside that is responsible for delivering care on a 24 hours a day, 365 days a year basis. Therefore, this text book devoted entirely to the topic of pressure area care for student and newly qualified nurses is long overdue. It is imperative that this aspect of care that crosses all care settings, affecting patients of any age and with many disease processes, is familiar to every practicing nurse wherever they chose to deliver care.

Many of the concepts discussed rely on good assessment techniques – the cornerstone of all care. Yet equally, many of these assessment and measurement tools are misunderstood and badly used in practice. The reflective approach to reading and practice taken in this text should encourage the student and novice nurse to take time out and review what they see, linking their theoretical knowledge to clinical practice. This should stimulate them to question what they see happening in day-to-day practice and start to implement high-quality, patient-focussed pressure area care. The focus on the role of the multidisciplinary team, particularly highlighting their roles, is so important in this speciality. It will hopefully produce a flurry of new practitioners to champion the cause of preventing pressure ulcers, working in partnership with both their colleagues from other disciplines but, more importantly, with the patient.

Jacqui Fletcher
Deputy Recorder EPUAP
Principal Lecturer Tissue Viability
University of Hertfordshire

Preface

This book has been written initially for student nurses and newly qualified practitioners who have an interest in pressure area care. I have aimed to offer you an overview of issues relating to pressure area care in a basic, easy-to-understand fashion. I originally developed my own personal interest in pressure care as a qualified practitioner working in an orthopaedic environment. During that time I came to appreciate that pressure ulcers are not a problem exclusively related to the older person, but can, indeed, affect any age group. I agreed to edit this book as I believe this is an area of nursing that every student, unqualified and qualified nurse will come across at some time during their career and that we should all be aware of the principles and concepts related to preventing and treating pressure ulcers.

As with all areas in nursing, principles, guidelines and concepts change over the years. It is, therefore, important that you ensure that you keep yourselves updated and read publications relevant to pressure area care and tissue viability. A good source of information is the Internet, where you can access up-to-date publications, for example, the Department of Health Website and the Tissue Viability Society. Remember that you are responsible for your own learning and as qualified practitioners you are accountable for your own practices. It is imperative that your practices are evidence based and, if questioned, you can offer a rationale for your choice of treatment and plan of care. I should mention here that at the present time the Nursing and Midwifery Council (NMC) are discussing the regulation of Health Care Assistants. If this is successful, then not only will it be the qualified staff who are accountable for their actions, but also the unqualified staff.

Acknowledgements

I would like to thank Duncan Mitchell, Lillian Neville and Melanie Stephens for their contributions to this book, and to the School of Nursing for supporting me in completing this text.

I would also like to thank the European Pressure Ulcer Advisory Panel (EPUAP), Elsevier Science, Quay Books, the Royal College of Nursing, the Department of Health and the National Institute for Clinical Excellence (NICE) for granting me permission to reproduce their material. It should be made clear that the NICE material is subject to copyright and any permission requests should be directed to the Communications Programme Director at NICE: www.nice.org.uk

The information that I have supplied in Appendix Three, from the *Essence of Care*, is also subject to copyright. If you need to reproduce any of this information you will be required to obtain a 'click user licence'. Advice on how to obtain a licence is contained on the HMSO website. Crown copyright material is reproduced with the permission of the Controller of HMSO and the Queen's Printer for Scotland.

Thanks also need to go to Benjamin Hepworth who kindly agreed to provide the illustrations for this text.

Contributors

Dr Duncan Mitchell
(contributor to Chapter 8)

RN (LD), Cert Ed, BA (Hons),
MA, PhD
Senior Lecturer
School of Nursing
University of Salford
Salford

Lillian Neville
(contributor to Chapter 8)

RGN, RNT, Cert Ed, MA
Senior Lecturer in Nursing
School of Nursing
University of Salford
Salford

Melanie Stephens
(contributor to Chapter 9)

RGN, BSc (Hons)
Lecturer in Nursing
School of Nursing
University of Salford
Salford

Introduction

HOW TO USE THIS BOOK

This book is designed to develop the knowledge of practitioners who have an interest in pressure area care. It will not give you all the answers to issues relevant to pressure area care. I hope that it will give you the enthusiasm to seek out further information and use up-to-date evidence to support your practice in the clinical areas and, where appropriate, to question practices. What it does aim to achieve is to give you an insight into the concepts and issues surrounding pressure area care.

Layout

The book contains ten chapters, three appendices and a glossary of terms. The appendices present you with additional information. Appendix One provides you with direction of why and how you search the literature to supplement your knowledge and increase your information base: it also presents a box of databases that may be useful for you when you are searching for further evidence or research to support your studies. Appendix Two presents you with the National Institute of Clinical Excellence (NICE) guidelines for pressure ulcer prevention (Clinical Guideline 7). Appendix Three presents you with the Department of Health's pressure ulcer recommendations from the *Essence of Care* document. I would recommend that you read the appendices in conjunction with the book, to help you understand the content of the NICE and Department of Health guidelines regarding pressure ulcer prevention and care.

I have included a glossary of terms from the book that I think will be helpful for you in understanding certain terminology used in this book.

Chapters

At the end of each chapter you will find a section that offers you the opportunity to reflect upon your newly acquired knowledge base. In addition, Chapters Two to Nine include a scenario to consolidate what you have learnt. This will help you to assess your knowledge base and will give you the opportunity to link the theory learnt, to the clinical areas where you will meet patients who are at risk of, or who already have developed a pressure ulcer. I believe that it is important that you re-evaluate your knowledge base following each chapter, to ensure that you have understood the information and concepts presented to you. By reflecting on your new knowledge base you will be able to assess any further individual learning needs you may have.

Why reflect?

As students and qualified practitioners we are encouraged to reflect on our practices. The concept of reflection is as important with education. When we learn something new we should take time to think about what we have learnt and how this will affect our practice in the future. I have therefore included a section for you to reflect at the end of each chapter. Schön (1983) distinguishes between the effective and the ineffective practitioner. He identifies the former as being able to recognise and explore confusing or unique events that occur during practice, and the latter being confined to repetitive and routine practice, neglecting opportunities to think about what we are doing. This description may be related to education as well as practice, in that, if you do not continue to develop your knowledge base and use that new found knowledge in practice, you will confine yourself to ritualistic practice. You should be continually striving to seek out new knowledge and evidence that underpins your practice, ensuring that you are administering the most effective and safe practices to your patients. In addition, you should be sharing your knowledge with others and questioning others when you are unsure as to why procedures are being carried out. To do this efficiently you need to reflect on your own education needs and maintain evidence-based practice.

Why complete a scenario?

The scenarios are devised to allow you to assess the patients' needs in a holistic manner rather than simply concentrating on pressure area care. They should help you to consolidate your knowledge after reading each chapter. Following each scenario I have provided you with some tips, relating to information that you may have gathered while working through it. The list is not exhaustive but will provide you with some ideas and will allow you to consider the thoughts you had. Do not worry if you have not considered all the ideas that I may have presented to you, simply go away and look them up to develop your own knowledge base. Remember, that you may have gathered far more information than I have suggested!

Tips on completing the scenario

Look at the information you have been presented with and consider the patient as a whole, rather than concentrating solely on pressure area care. Remember that the patients you will nurse in clinical areas will have their care assessed, planned, implemented and evaluated in a holistic manner. It is important that you take this into account when learning the underpinning knowledge, as it will help you to link theory to practice. You may want to write down all your initial ideas of which areas require exploration and then subdivide the information you require into four areas:

Care delivery

Here you may decide which care interventions are required for your patient and how you will assess and plan that care. Within this area it may be useful to review your knowledge on the anatomy and physiology of the condition your patient has presented with, to allow you to be able to administer effective and safe nursing care.

Care management

Here you may decide how you will manage that plan of care, for example, when will you reevaluate, which assessment tools will you use, will you involve other members of the interdisciplinary team in the care being delivered?

Professional and ethical

Here you will think about any legal or ethical aspects you may have to consider. You may also want to examine any policies, protocols, guidelines or Government papers that have been produced, which are relevant to your patients' care and reflect upon how they impact on the clinical care.

Professional and personal development

Here you may want to extend your own knowledge base further in an area that you have an interest in. This will be different for everyone.

It is worth remembering that you can also ask clinical staff or your tutors within the school of nursing for information or guidance on where to seek out the information. I hope you enjoy the scenarios and happy information gathering!

Overview of Appendix 3 (*Essence of Care*) and guidance for use

The following section offers you a brief overview of how to use the *Essence of Care* document. At the start of the document you will find a section entitled 'using the tool' that explains clearly how you should use the document and the sections inside it.

The eight aspects of care

The *Essence of Care* document (DoH, 2001) is described as a practical toolkit for nurses and others. It is divided into eight aspects of care covering the following topics:

- Principles of self-care
- Food and nutrition
- Personal and oral hygiene
- Continence and bladder and bowel care
- Pressure ulcers
- Record keeping
- Safety of clients/patients with mental health needs in acute mental health and general hospital settings
- Privacy and dignity

The *Essence of Care* document has been designed to help to improve quality and to contribute to clinical governance initiatives at a local level. It is a benchmarking activity that helps practitioners to take a structured approach to sharing and comparing practice, enabling them to identify the best and to develop action plans to remedy poor practice (DoH, 2001, p. 8). The approach involves the identification of patient focused best practice in aspects of care that are crucial to the quality of care received by the patient.

Benchmarking

Each of the benchmarking tools in the sections of the document follows the same format. These are presented below and reproduced with kind permission from the Controller of HMSO and the Queen's Printer for Scotland.

(1) An overall statement, which expresses what patients/ clients/consumers want from care (*patient/client focused outcome*).

(2) Suggested *indicators* or *information* that is currently gathered, which may indicate action is required to improve poor practice or that good practice exists which should be shared with others.

(3) Elements of practice that support the attainment of the patient/client focused outcome (*factors*).

(4) Key sources: policies, documents, references and the evidence base used in compilation.

(5) Patient/client focused best practice in each of the factors, the *benchmark*, which is placed at the extreme right of a series of statements and allotted an A score.

(6) A scoring continuum for each factor. These statements guide practitioners in awarding their own practice a score, and provide stepping stones for practitioners to consider taking, in order to achieve best practice.

A diagrammatic presentation of benchmark statements is shown here.

Factor 1

Worst practice statement	Statements of practice that step towards best practice			Best practice statement
[E]	D	C	B	[A]

(7) Finally, there is space for the identification of evidence that comparison group members agree would justify an A score in their particular area of practice (for like to like comparison).

(8) Statements around best practice were identified by patients/clients, consumers and professionals and are attached to help stimulate comparison group discussions.

After each benchmark the pack contains examples of documentation to support the use of the benchmarking tool:

- Comparison group information
- Scoring sheet

- Comparison group collated scores
- Action planned to develop practice

What you will see when you read the aspect of care relevant to your patient care

When you obtain a copy of the *Essence of Care*, or refer to Appendix Three, you will note that each aspect of care is presented in the same format, as identified above. The beginning of each section will give you a definition of the aspect of care to be discussed. This will be followed by the agreed patient/client focused outcome and then the indicators/information that highlights concerns, which may trigger the need for the benchmarking activity. In relation to pressure ulcers, the document has identified nine factors that each practitioner needs to undertake when caring for their patient. These are listed below:

(1) Screening/assessment
(2) Who undertakes the assessment?
(3) Informing patients/clients/carers (prevention and treatment)
(4) Individualised plan for prevention and treatment of pressure ulcers
(5) Pressure ulcer prevention – repositioning
(6) Pressure ulcer prevention – redistributing support surfaces
(7) Pressure ulcer prevention – availability of resources, equipment
(8) Implementation of individualised plan
(9) Evaluation of interventions by a registered practitioner

You will see that beside each identified factor is the benchmark for best practice (Appendix Three). Each factor is then discussed in detail, highlighting the worst practice statement and best practice statement. All users should be aiming to achieve the best practice statement. You will then be asked to provide the evidence to support your own practices at local level. This will include documenting any policies, procedures or guidelines that may be in use; education available for the staff; resources; the integration of the multidisciplinary team in caring for the patients and other examples that may be relevant (Appendix Three). You will then be presented with a number of statements that should stimulate discussion around best practice.

Following discussion of all the factors there is space for the comparison group to document their collated scores and to justify why they have reached those scores. When the group has discussed their scores and agreed where, in the continuum, the care on their unit is, an action plan is presented for the group to complete. Here the group is expected to agree on the action required to enable the best practice statement to be achieved, with dates and names of practitioners who are responsible for ensuring this is completed. The document also encourages practitioners to reflect upon the process.

I suggest that you refer to Appendix Three prior to reading this book, as the document is referred to within the chapters. If you have any questions relating to the content of the *Essence of Care* then please ask for advice and clarification from either a clinical practitioner or a member of the clinical ward staff. The Crown copyright material is reproduced with the permission of the Controller of HMSO and the Queen's Printer for Scotland.

REFERENCE

Department of Health (2001) *The Essence of Care – patient-focused benchmarking for health care practitioners.* Department of Health, London.
Schön, D. A. (1983) *The Reflective Practitioner: How Professionals Think in Action.* Arena, Aldershot.

The Importance of Effective Pressure Area Care

1

INTRODUCTION

This chapter will briefly introduce the history of pressure area care, allowing you an insight into this exciting area of nursing that tends to encompass every speciality. It will also highlight the importance of preventing the development of pressure ulcers and possessing the underpinning knowledge for your interventions. The chapter will also discuss the importance of maintaining quality and will identify examples of quality tools that you may witness in practice. You may find it beneficial to discuss practices with the tissue viability specialist based within your area of work, who will be able to explain and define care interventions. It may now be appropriate for you to refer to Appendix Two that presents the NICE guidelines (2003) regarding pressure ulcer prevention and Appendix Three that refers to the *Essence of Care* (DoH, 2001) guidance for pressure ulcers.

Appendix One explains how and why you should search the literature to gain information and offers some examples of useful databases.

LEARNING OBJECTIVES

By the end of this chapter the reader will be enabled to:

❏ Identify the financial costs associated with pressure ulcer development
❏ Briefly discuss the history of wound care
❏ Identify the human suffering associated with pressure ulcer development

❑ Discuss the concept of evidence-based practice
❑ Discuss the importance of maintaining quality

Cost of pressure ulcers

Pressure ulcers are an unpleasant complication of illness or disability. They can be defined as: ulceration of the skin following disruption of the blood supply due to pressure, friction or shear, or a combination of all of these factors (Dealey, 1994). What must be remembered is not only the human suffering that pressure ulcers cause to the individual, but also the monetary cost. The financial costs associated with the treatment of pressure ulcers have become a concern for all involved, including the Government, who, in the *Health of the Nation* document, set targets to reduce the prevalence by between 5% and 10%. Reid and Morison (1994) reviewed the literature pertaining to the prevalence of pressure ulcers inpatients, and concluded that the rate still lay between 6% and 14%, with other writers claiming that the figure continues to be much higher than this.

The Department of Health (1992, 1993) estimated the cost to the NHS of pressure ulcers at between £60 million and £321 million, with Hibbs (1990) stating that the treatment of a pressure ulcer that has damaged all the layers of the skin is £26 000, whereas, Collier (1999) has further increased this estimate to be at £40 000. Clough (1994) assessed the costs of treating pressure ulcers in an intensive care unit, calculating the cost to be £150 per patient per day to prevent pressure ulcers, that rose to £320 to treat them. The cost of treatment is not only the cost incurred by the hospital, but also the cost of litigation, which has become more popular over the last few years.

Therefore, the need for education for all professionals involved in pressure area care and the ability to utilise the available resources in an effective and efficient manner remains important.

History of pressure area care

Pressure ulcers are by no means new phenomena. They were found on bodies of Egyptian mummies, with Thompson (1961) recording the discovery of pressure ulcers on the body of a priestess of Amen of the XXIth Dynasty (2050–1800 BC), stating that they were found to be carefully covered with pieces of soft leather before embalming, probably in an attempt to restore physical integrity. In 1593, Fabricius Hilanus, a surgeon from the Netherlands, described the clinical characteristics of pressure ulcers. He claimed that external natural and internal supernatural factors were causes, as well as the interruption in the supply of the 'pneuma', blood and nutrients (Defloor, 1999). During the sixteenth century, Ambrose Pare, a French surgeon, treated war injuries and pressure ulcers. Interestingly, his recommendations remain relevant today, with his suggestion that healthy nutrition, curing underlying illness, pressure relief, psychological support, surgical treatment and dressings were all important aspects in the prevention and treatment of pressure ulcers (Levine, 1992).

In 1879, Charcot, a neurologist, suggested that pressure ulcers in patients with a spinal injury were inevitable and that doctors could do nothing about them, as they were a result of neurogenic trophic factors. By 1938, it was suggested that the unstable scar of a healed pressure ulcer be replaced with flap tissue, and in 1947 it was being recommended that the bony prominences were excised and the exposed bone padded with local fascia or muscle fascia flaps.

The role of nurses in the prevention of pressure ulcers

It was in 1860 that Florence Nightingale recognised the responsibility of nurses in the prevention of pressure ulcers and she maintained that they could be prevented by good nursing care, and that if a patient did develop a pressure ulcer it was the fault of poor nursing care rather than the disease. This idea is often replicated today, with many nurses feeling dreadful guilt if their patient develops a pressure ulcer. It is only recently that the importance of an interdisciplinary approach to the prevention and treatment of pressure ulcers has been acknowledged with us seeing regular prevalence and incidence studies being carried out in care settings to try to ascertain the depth of the problem and to find a solution.

The creation of the Tissue Viability Society in 1980 helped to promote the importance of an interdisciplinary approach and raised the awareness of medical staff that they, too, should participate in prevention and treatment strategies. Unfortunately, medical schools still do not view this area of medicine as a priority in the training of medical staff and the students receive very little education on the subject, often relying on nursing staff to educate them when they are in clinical practice.

Ideas regarding the prevention and treatment of pressures ulcers have changed over the years. What has remained constant is the understanding that relief of pressure from the vulnerable areas is required, to the extent that until the mid 1980s many areas carried out a 'back round'. The 'back round' involved nurses washing and massaging the pressure areas of bedfast patients and applying a range of lotions, creams, powder, oils and spirits in an attempt to prevent breakdown of the skin. If a pressure ulcer were to occur then treatments varied. They included: lying the patient on their side to reduce pressure and administering oxygen, by placing an oxygen mask over the ulcer to maintain a dry environment; placing a dressing of egg white over the affected area, with the thought that it would heal the ulcer due to the protein content of the egg. Thankfully, staff now accept the concept of maintaining a moist wound-healing environment (Winter, 1962) and the dressings used reflect this. The use of appropriate dressings for the treatment of a pressure ulcer is discussed in detail in Chapter Seven.

THE IMPORTANCE OF EFFECTIVE PRESSURE AREA CARE

The importance of preventing and treating pressure ulcers is now a worldwide concern for all health professionals. The European Pressure Ulcer Advisory Panel (EPUAP) was set up to deal with the problem at a European level in 1997 and continues to offer recommendations and guidelines today.

The Human Rights Act (1998) saw the publication of various articles and, according to Dimond (2003), Articles 2 and 3 appear to relate directly to the issue of tissue viability. Article 2 states that law shall protect everyone's right to life. In some cases pressure ulcers and tissue damage are so severe that they can cause the death of a patient. In such cases it could be argued that the failure to provide a proper standard of care has led to the death of a patient and is, therefore, a breach of Article 2. Article 3 gives a right not to be subjected to torture or to inhumane or degrading treatment or punishment. In the worst-case scenario failure to prevent the occurrence of tissue breakdown may be viewed as inhuman or degrading treatment. Trusts and healthcare personnel, therefore, have a duty to provide reasonable health services, and failures to fulfil this duty by causing pressure ulcers may be seen as breach of Article 3.

Evidence-based practice

It is important that evidence-based practice is maintained when implementing care to prevent or treat pressure ulcer development. DiCenso *et al.* (1998) argue that in practising evidence-based nursing a nurse has to decide whether the evidence is relevant for that particular patient. The nurse should then consider the risks and benefits of alternative treatments and should take into account the individu ' ˜˜ods of each patient, including comorbid conditions and
It is important that your initial assessment of ˀ
needs is comprehensive and that you have d˸
explained to the patient the plan of care ˀ   ᴑ

implement and your reasons for this decision, ensuring that the patient is able to give you their informed consent. The Department of Health (2001) asserts that all patients' records must demonstrate that their care follows evidence-based guidance or supporting documents describing best practice.

Evidence may be obtained from a variety of sources and these include:

- Research
- Experiential evidence
- Evidence from specialists
- Policies

Essentially, evidence-based practice seeks to direct health professionals towards interventions that provide real benefits for the patients and will enable practitioners to administer the best possible care to their patients, helping to maintain and develop standards. Boynton (2001) supports this idea of evidence-based practice by arguing that the development, implementation and maintenance of evidence-based practice positively affect structure, process and patient care outcomes.

Quality issues

The Department of Health (1999) has stated that it is for every nurse, midwife and health visitor to strive for quality improvement in all aspects of practice. This statement has been directly related to the prevention of pressure ulcers through the implementation of various documents and guidelines that include:

- *Pressure Sores: a Key Quality Indicator* (DoH, 1993)
- *Making a Difference. A Strategy for Nursing* (DoH, 1999)
- *Essence of Care: Patient-Focused Benchmarking for Health Care Practitioners* (DoH 2001)
- *Pressure Ulcer Risk Assessment and Prevention Guidelines* (NICE, 2001)

The Nursing and Midwifery Council

As a registered nurse, midwife or health visitor you must maintain your professional knowledge and competence. The Nursing and Midwifery Council (NMC) have stated in the *Code of Professional Conduct* (2002) that you must keep your knowledge and skills up to date throughout your working life and that to practice competently you must:

'Possess the knowledge, skills and abilities required for lawful, safe and effective practice without direct supervision. You must acknowledge the limits of your professional competence and only undertake practice and accept responsibilities for those activities in which you are competent'

(NMC, 6.1, 6.2 2002).

In addition, the NMC (2002, 6.5) quite clearly state that you have a responsibility to deliver evidence-based care and where applicable, care that is research based. It is, therefore, unmistakable that as a registered nurse, midwife or health visitor it is your own professional responsibility to maintain your knowledge and standards. As a student nurse you should be aware of the *Code of Professional Conduct* and what it entails, since you are training to become a qualified practitioner who will be required to adhere by this document.

In relation to student nurses the NMC (2002) state that:

'As a pre-registration student, you are never professionally accountable in the way that you will be after you come to register with the NMC. This means that you can never be called to account for your actions or omissions by the NMC.'

However, they do state that:

'This does not mean, that you can never be called to account by your university or by the law for the consequences of your actions or omissions as a pre-registration student.'

The NMC guide for students of nursing and midwifery (NMC, 2002) quite clearly identifies that as a student nurse you must also ensure that you, too, are competent to undertake a task through education and a strong knowledge base. Once again, if you are unsure as to how you should undertake a procedure, do *not* do it and ask for supervision or to observe it being undertaken by a competent practitioner.

CONCLUSION

This chapter has given you an overview of the importance of effective pressure area care and the history of wound care. The concept of effective pressure area care will be referred to throughout this book and the issues built upon. What is important to remember is that the prevention and treatment of pressure ulcers is not a new phenomenon and that any patient, regardless of age, sex, admitting condition or weight, is prone to developing pressure ulcers. Therefore, as healthcare professionals, we all have a responsibility to help prevent their development and to prevent the human suffering that can occur. Furthermore, the NMC supports the need for all qualified practitioners to maintain their education and knowledge base to administer care based upon the best available evidence.

REFERENCES

Boynton, P. R. (2001) Quality assurance and audit. In: *The Prevention and Treatment of Pressure Ulcers*, (ed. Morison, M. J.). Mosby, London.

Clough, N. P. (1994) The cost of pressure area management in an intensive care unit. *Journal of Wound Care*, **3**, (1), 33–5.

Collier, M. (1999) Pressure ulcer development and principles for prevention. In: *Wound Management: Theory and Practice* (eds Glover, D. & Miller, M.), pp. 84–95. EMAP, London.

Dealey, C. (1994) *The Care of Wounds*. Blackwell Scientific Publications, Oxford.

Defloor, T. (1999) The risk of pressure sores: a conceptual scheme. *Journal of Clinical Nursing*, **8**, 206–16.

Department of Health (1992) *The Health of the Nation.* HMSO, London.

Department of Health (1993) *Pressure Sores: a Key Quality Indicator.* HMSO, London.

Department of Health (1999) *Making a Difference. Strategy for Nursing.* Department of Health Publications, London.

Department of Health (2001) *Essence of Care. Patient-focused Benchmarking for Health Care Practitioners.* Department of Health, London.

DiCenso, A., Cullum, N. & Ciliska, D. (1998) Implementing evidence-based nursing: some misconceptions. *Evidence-Based Nursing,* **1** (2), 38–40.

Dimond, B. (2003) Pressure ulcers and litigation. *Nursing Times: Wound Care Supplement,* **99** (5).

Hibbs, P. (1990) The economics of pressure sores. In: *Pressure Sores: Clinical Practice and Scientific Approach* (ed. Bader, D.), pp. 35–42. Macmillan, London.

HMSO (1998) The Human Rights Act www.hmso.gov.uk/acts/ act1998 accessed 31 March 2003.

Levine, J. M. (1992) Historical notes on pressure ulcers: the cure of Ambrose Pare. *Decubitus,* **5**, 23–6.

Morrell, C. & Harvey, G. (1999) *The Clinical Audit Handbook. Improving the Quality of Health Care.* Baillière Tindall, London.

National Institute for Clinical Excellence (2001) Pressure ulcer risk management and prevention. *Inherited Clinical Guideline B.* National Institute for Clinical Excellence, London.

National Institute for Clinical Excellence (2003) *Pressure Ulcer Prevention. Pressure Ulcer Risk Assessment and Prevention; Including the Use of Pressure-relieving Devices (Beds, Mattresses and Overlays) for the Prevention of Pressure Ulcers in Primary and Secondary Care.* NICE Clinical guideline No 7. National Institute for Clinical Excellence, London. Available from: www.nice.org.uk

Nursing and Midwifery Council (2002) *An NMC Guide for Students of Nursing and Midwifery.* Nursing and Midwifery Council, London.

Nursing and Midwifery Council (2002) *Code of Professional Conduct.* Nursing and Midwifery Council, London.

Reid, J. & Morison, M. (1994) Classification of pressure sore severity. *Nursing Times,* **90** (20), 46–50.

Royal College of Nursing (2001) *A Guide for Patients and Their Carers: Working Together to Prevent Pressure Ulcer.* Royal College of Nursing, London.

Royal College of Nursing (2001) *Clinical Practice Guidelines: Pressure Ulcer Risk Assessment and Prevention. Recommendations 2001.* Royal College of Nursing, London.

Thompson, J. (1961) Pathological changes in mummies. *Proceedings of the Royal Society of Medicine*, **54**, 409–15.

Winter, G. D. (1962) Formation of scab and the rate of epithelialisation of superficial wounds in the skin of the domestic pig. *Nature*, **193**, 293–4.

Anatomy and Physiology of the Skin and the Wound Healing Process

2

INTRODUCTION

This chapter will identify and discuss the pathophysiology and aetiology of pressure ulcers, followed by a description of the wound healing process. Finally, you will be asked to reflect upon your knowledge base and complete a scenario related to the information in the chapter.

LEARNING OBJECTIVES

By the end of this chapter the reader will be enabled to:

❏ Identify the pathophysiology of pressure ulcers
❏ Describe the anatomy and physiology of the skin
❏ Discuss the aetiology of pressure ulcers
❏ Describe the wound healing process

Why is it important to develop your knowledge?

Knowledge of the epidemiology of pressure ulcers, anatomy and physiology of the skin, and causative factors of the development of pressure ulcers are the first, probably most important step, any practitioner must undertake in the quest to meet the challenge in their prevention. It is important that all practitioners are aware of the pathophysiology and aetiology of pressure ulcers and mechanisms to prevent pressure ulcer development.

Pathophysiology and aetiology of pressure ulcers

Anatomy of the skin

Tissues involved in pressure ulcer development are the skin, subcutaneous fat, deep fascia, muscle and bone. The skin is the largest organ of the body; in adults the skin covers an area of about two square metres, and weighs 4.5–5 kg; it ranges in thickness from 0.5 to 4.0 mm depending on location. The skin forms a protective barrier around the body; indeed, it is alive, casting off old cells and renewing itself, often reflecting the status of the body's health.

Its external environment is equipped with sensors to monitor changes in external physical conditions. The receptor cells show a wide variation in structure and location: some lie superficially and are sensitive to light or heat touch; others are deeply placed and activated only by severe pressure (Vannini & Pogliani, 1999). It is a dynamic structure in which cellular replacement and modification in response to local need is a continual process throughout life. It is relatively resistant to water, chemicals and bacteria, and provides some protection for the body against mechanical damage. Structurally the skin is a layered organ containing three layers:

- The epidermis
- The dermis
- Subcutaneous tissue

(Barton & Barton, 1981)

The word 'dermis' comes from the Greek word for skin, with the Greek word 'epi' meaning 'over'. Thus, when the words 'epi' and 'dermis' are added together they form the word 'epidermis', translating as the outer layer of the skin.

Figure 2.1 shows a basic representation of the structure of the skin.

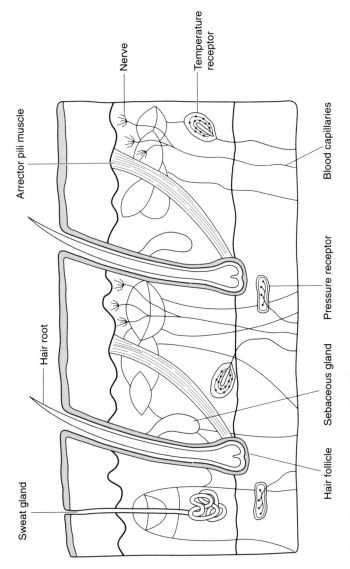

Arrector pili muscle

Nerve

Temperature receptor

Blood capillaries

Hair root

Pressure receptor

Sebaceous gland

Sweat gland

Hair follicle

Fig. 2.1 Diagram of the structure of the skin.

Epidermis

The epidermis consists mainly of stratified squamous epithelium (keratinocytes) and a small number of melanocytes (for melanin synthesis), Langerhans cells (antigen-presenting cells) and Merkel cells (for neuroendocrine function). They are placed side by side and arranged one above the other in several layers. The squamous epithelium cells are arranged in four layers:

- The stratum corneum
- The granular layer
- The stratum spinosum
- The stratum germinativum (or basal layer)

The stratum corneum layer consists of cells, which have no nuclei or cytoplasmic organelles, contain little water, are tightly packed and provide a physical barrier against water, bacteria and chemicals. The cells are constantly being shed and replaced by cells from deeper layers. The basement membrane separates the basal cells from the underlying dermis and the basal cells are attached to the membrane by structures known as hemidesmosomes. This basal lamina region consists of four zones:

- The plasma membrane of the epidermal cells, which contain hemidesmosomes
- An electron-lucent area (lamina lucida), which contains the protein lamina
- An electron-dense area (lamina densa), consisting of type IV collagen
- Extensions of the lamina densa, providing attachments to the underlying dermis (Woolf, 1998)

There are some nerve cells in the epidermis, but there are no blood vessels. It contains melanin that is responsible for the colour of skin, suntan and freckles.

Dermis

The dermis is the inner and thicker layer of the skin, which lies beneath the epidermis and consists of two layers:

- The papillary dermis, which is configured in a series of papillae separated by projections of the epidermis known as rete pegs (Scales, 1990).
- The reticular dermis, which is beneath an imaginary line joining the tips of the rete pegs and consists of thick collagen bundles orientated parallel to the overlying epidermis (Woolf, 1998).

The dermis is highly vascular and well supplied with sensory receptors to pain, temperature and touch. It contains blood capillaries, sebaceous glands, hair follicles and lymphatic capillaries. A matrix of collagen and elastin support these structures. The upper layer of the dermis presents as cobbled, valleyed and meshed areas with the pitted undersurface of the epidermis binding the two together. These ridges are arranged in regular curved rows and are as unique to the individual as fingerprints. Ducts of sweat glands surface through these ridges to give a non-skid surface to hands and feet, enabling us to pick up small objects and perform delicate manipulations. Into this upper layer of the dermis come thousands of capillaries, the small blood vessels that bring food and oxygen to the cells and remove waste. The inner layer is strong and elastic, containing nerve fibres, hair follicles, oil and sweat glands, muscular elements and receptor organs for sensations of:

- Touch
- Pain
- Heat and cold

Deeper in the dermis are the roots of the skin glands and hair, as well as more blood and lymph vessels, nerves and larger and tougher fibres (www.caretechlabs.com). Note that the dermis cannot regenerate if destroyed, that is to say, it heals by secondary intention with the formation of granulation tissue, which is then replaced by scar tissue.

Subcutaneous layer
A subcutaneous layer separates the dermis from the deeper structures of the deep fascia, muscle and bone. Thickness of the layer varies, dependent upon the presence of fat cells, which provide mobility to skin and padding to disperse pressure. The fat cells are arranged in lobules, which are separated by bands of connective tissue known as interlobular septa (Woolf, 1998).

Deep fascia
The deep fascia is a dense, essentially avascular, inelastic membrane, which covers muscle and muscle groups, and over bony prominences may merge with the outer layer of the bone. It is resistant to pressure and is the last line of protection of vulnerable muscle tissue (Morison, 2001). See figure 2.1.

Accessory organs of the skin
The accessory organs of the skin are the skin glands, the hair and the nails.

Skin glands
There are two types of skin glands:

- Ones that pour out sweat
- Ones that secrete oil

Sweat glands
There are approximately two million sweat glands found all over the body. Most are found on the forehead, face, palms, soles, the groin and the body surface. These glands give off a

small amount of waste material but their main function is to regulate body heat.

Sebaceous glands
These glands produce oil and fats, and generally open into the hair follicle producing sebum. The sebum penetrates into the hair follicle and works its way to the surface, where it spreads a thin film to lubricate the hair shaft and the horny layers of the skin. The lubricant also helps to prevent excessive evaporation and absorption of water and excess heat loss. The sebum plays an important role in maintaining the normal acidity of the skin, keeping the skin soft and supple. The surface of normal healthy skin is slightly acid in reaction; if there should be a change towards alkalinity the skin is thought to become more susceptible to fungal infection.

Hair
Pushing a group of cells upwards at its base, and in the process becoming keratinised, develops hair. The part of the hair that is visible is the shaft, with the root being embedded in the dermis. The root alongside its covering forms the hair follicle, which has a loop of capillaries enclosed in connective tissue called the hair papilla. The cluster of epithelial cells lying over the papilla are reproduced and eventually form the shaft; as long as these cells remain alive hair will regenerate. The hair is kept soft by sebaceous glands that secrete varying amounts of oily sebum into the follicle near the surface of the skin. Attached to these follicles are the erector pili muscles, which make the hair stand on end when they contract.

Figure 2.2 represents a cross-section of the skin.

Physiology of the skin
The skin has several functions:

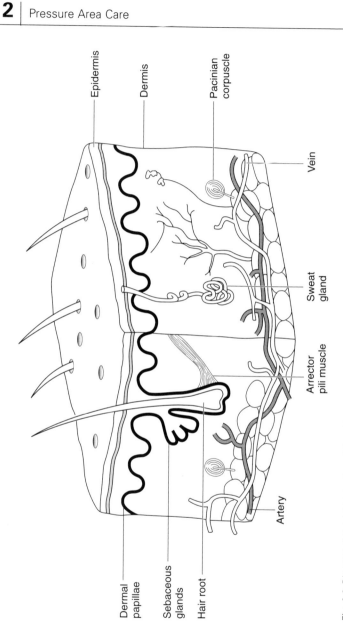

Epidermis

Dermis

Pacinian corpuscle

Vein

Sweat gland

Arrector pili muscle

Artery

Dermal papillae

Sebaceous glands

Hair root

Fig. 2.2 Diagram of the cross-section of the skin.

(1) **Regulation of body temperature**   In response to a high environment of temperature the evaporation of sweat from the skin surface helps to lower an elevated body temperature to normal. Alternatively, in response to low body temperature the production of sweat is decreased to aid in the conservation of heat.

(2) **Protection**   The skin covers the body, providing a protective barrier that protects the underlying tissues from abrasions, bacterial invasion, dehydration and ultraviolet radiation.

(3) **Sensation**   The skin contains many nerve endings and receptors that detect stimuli related to touch, pressure, pain and temperature.

(4) **Excretion**   In addition to removing heat and some water from the body, sweat also acts as the vehicle for excretion of a small amount of salts and several organic compounds.

(5) **Immunity**   Certain cells of the epidermis are important components of the immune system.

(6) **Blood reservoir**   The dermis of the skin houses extensive networks of blood vessels that carry 8–10% of the total blood flow in a resting adult. In moderate exercise skin blood flow may increase, which helps dispel heat from the body. During hard exercise the skin blood vessels constrict and more blood is able to flow to the contracting muscles.

(7) **Synthesis of vitamin D**   Vitamin D synthesis begins with activation of a precursor molecule in the skin by ultraviolet rays in the sunlight. Enzymes in the liver and kidneys then modify the molecule, finally producing calcitriol, which is the most active form of Vitamin D. Calcitriol, contributes to the homeostasis of body fluids by aiding absorption of calcium in foods.

(adapted from Tortora & Grabowski, 1999)

A healthy blood supply is required for the skin's survival with the skin receiving up to one third of the body's circulating blood. A network of vascular and lymph vessels ensure the necessary nutrients and oxygen are supplied to support cell metabolism and epidermal mitosis, with the blood flow facilitating temperature regulation and the removal of waste products from the skin. The arteries supporting the skin pierce the deep fascia and form a network of arterioles in the subcutaneous tissues, with capillary branches supplying the hair follicles and sebaceous and sweat glands within the dermis. The arterioles are highly muscular, which enables them to change their diameter and to branch into a network of metarterioles that have a structure midway between arterioles and capillaries. They do not have a continuous muscle coat, but smooth muscle fibres encircle the blood vessel at intermediate points (Guyton, 1992).

The metarterioles further subdivide into capillaries, some of which are large and are called preferential channels, and others, which are small and known as true capillaries. The smooth muscle cells at the origin of the capillaries act as precapillary sphincters and are important in the control of blood. The capillaries are composed of a single layer of highly permeable endothelial cells surrounded by a basement membrane. Between each endothelial cell is a small channel referred to as an intercellular cleft, and within the endothelial cells are plasmalemmal vesicles. These structures are important in the exchange of nutrients and other substances between the blood and interstitial fluid (Guyton, 1992).

An important characteristic of the vascular system is the ability of each tissue to control local blood flow in proportion to need. Various acute and long-term auto-regulatory mechanisms are evident to ensure that blood flow is directly related to local tissue demand.

Observation of the microcirculation by microscope reveals that there is an intermittent ebb and flow through the capillary network controlled by the opening and closing of the metarterioles and precapillary sphincters, known as vasomotion (Guyton, 1992). An interplay of osmotic and hydrostatic pressures of plasma and interstitial fluid determine capillary permeability and reabsorption, as well as directly affecting the use of lymph vessels in removing proteins, large waste particles and excess fluid. The rapid flow of blood through the arteries and arterioles causes shear stress on the endothelial cells of the artery wall resulting in the release of endothelium derived relaxing factor (EDRF). The EDRF then relaxes the arterial muscle and the artery dilates, thus increasing the blood supply. In the long term, if blood flow continues excessively for days, weeks, or months, the arterial vessels enlarge.

Indeed, the size of the arterial vessels appear to readjust throughout life so that blood flow velocity is never great enough to cause an inordinate amount of blood flow resistance (Guyton, 1992). An acute increase or decrease in arterial blood pressure will result in a surge or reduction in blood flow through a tissue but within minutes an auto-regulatory mechanism readjusts flows to values of approximately three-quarters of the previous level. The resulting auto-regulation of blood flow ensures protection of capillaries from excessive pressure and maintains blood flow despite changes in arterial pressure. Over a period of time a long-term regulatory mechanism is apparent, with control established by changes in the vascularity of the tissue. Similarly, an auto-regulatory mechanism, known as the veni-arteriolar response, protects the microcirculation from increases in venous pressure.

Other mechanisms involved in the control of blood flow include nervous and humoral mechanisms, whereby various vasoconstrictor agents and vasodilator agents are released. Some result in systemic effects and others in localised changes to the tissue/organ blood flow (Guyton, 1992). When an external pressure is applied to the skin, for example, when sitting or lying in one position for a length of time, an auto-regulatory process allows the internal capillary pressure to rise accordingly, in response to the external load.

Wound healing process

Moist wound healing

As mentioned in the previous chapter, Winter (1962) explained the concept of moist healing. Moist wound healing is promoted to be the most effective way to heal a wound. He claimed that the epidermal cells could not migrate across a dry surface easily and that epidermal migration was much faster in moist wounds, as the cells did not have to negotiate a scab. A moist wound-healing environment encourages rehydration and autolysis and can help to remove dead tissue from the wound bed.

There are some types of wounds where moist wound healing is inappropriate. These include necrotic digits, where the necrosis is due to ischaemia. Clinicians believe that as infection is a high risk in these types of wounds, it is better to keep them dry. It is also worth seeking specialist advice regarding neuropathic and neuro/ischaemic diabetic ulcers. People with diabetes have a compromised healing mechanism and are more susceptible to infection; therefore, a moist healing environment may increase the potential risk of infection.

Types of wound healing

There are two types of wound healing. Primary intention occurs where the edges of the wound are brought together and held by methods such as sutures or staples. This is normally a surgical wound. They tend to heal quickly without complication. Secondary intention refers to those wounds that are left open and heal more slowly: these include pressure ulcers.

The process of wound healing can be divided into four phases:

(1) Vascular response or homeostasis
(2) Inflammation
(3) Proliferation
(4) Maturation

These phases do not occur in isolation, but with substantial overlap. The time taken for a wound to heal will vary between each individual and therefore a specific time limit cannot be attributed to the length of the process.

The vascular response

If damage to the skin affects more than the epidermis you will witness bleeding. The damaged ends of the blood vessels will constrict within seconds of the injury, to minimise the blood flow and to commence the blood clotting process, which is further developed by platelet aggregation and the release of growth factors necessary for wound repair. The blood clot, consisting of a fibrin mesh, will eventually become a scab that closes the wound and vasodilatation of the vessels begins.

Inflammation

This stage protects the body from further damage, dealing with toxins and killing bacteria. Phagocytosis commences, which is the ingestion of foreign material by the neutrophils and monocytes. Some of the monocytes will mature into macrophages that continue to clean the wound bed during the inflammatory stage. It is during this stage that you may observe erythema, heat, oedema, discomfort and functional disturbance around the wound area. These are due to an increase in blood flow and an accumulation of fluid in the soft tissues; they are a normal part of the inflammatory process and should not be confused with infection. This stage may last for up to four days, during which time the wound lacks tensile strength. If the wound is infected this stage may be prolonged. This phase is critical to the wound-healing process but some patients may be unable to produce this stage due to drug therapies, cancer or advanced age, and the wound will therefore not heal.

Proliferation

During this stage the wound begins to replace lost tissue and form collagen fibres that will give the wound its strength. The fibres support the capillary loops and new capillary buds that form the base for the new granulation tissue across the wound, promoting an increased supply of oxygen to the wound. This process is known as angiogenesis. Epithelial cells will then begin to migrate across the wound surface providing they have a moist environment and viable granulation tissue. Wounds that are granulating will appear bright red and be moist. As epithelialisation occurs the wound becomes a paler pink and less moist in appearance.

Maturation

This is the final stage of the wound-healing process and may continue for over twelve months from the initial injury. The wound regains its strength and function, but note that the wound never fully regains its pre-injury strength. During this stage scarring occurs.

Summary

The skin is the largest structure of the body. It provides protection from mechanical disruption, as do the tissues below. All tissues in the body are capable of healing and this occurs through two mechanisms:

- **Regeneration**   This is where damaged tissue is replaced by an identical replication of cells. In humans, complete regeneration is only possible in a limited number of cell types. For example, epithelial, liver and nerve cells.
- **Repair**   This is where damaged tissue is replaced by connective tissue, which then forms a scar. This is usually the main mechanism by which healing occurs (Flanagan, 1997).

The process of wound healing is divided into four phases: the vascular response; inflammation; proliferation and maturation. The phases tend to overlap and the time that the wound will spend in each stage is individual to each person.

CONCLUSION

This chapter has briefly described the anatomy and physiology of the skin and the wound-healing process. It is important that you understand these concepts when dealing with patients who are at risk of, or who have, an established pressure ulcer. There are numerous anatomy and physiology textbooks available if you wish to further develop your knowledge and understanding of these concepts.

SELF-ASSESSMENT

After reading this chapter you should now take some time to reassess your knowledge base.

Reflection

Take some time to reflect upon the knowledge you have gained and how you will implement it into your own practice.

What knowledge did I possess prior to reading this chapter?

What do I know now?

How will my practice change as a result of attaining this knowledge?

Do I need to discuss with anyone practices I have witnessed that are not evidence-based, in relation to my new knowledge?

If so, who will I speak to?

Scenario

Complete this scenario based upon the knowledge you now possess.

You are a third-year student nurse and have been asked by your mentor to deliver a teaching session to two first-year student nurses on the wound-healing process. You have decided that you will offer the students an overview of the anatomy and physiology of the skin and describe the wound healing process.

Tips on completing the scenario

Below is some information that you may have considered while working through the scenario. It is not an exhaustive list, but it will give you some guidance on the information you should have collected.

You should have revisited the anatomy and physiology of the skin and causes of pressure ulcer development.

You should have included the normal anatomy and physiology and drawn a diagram of the skin, showing the main structures of the skin. This will include highlighting that the skin is the largest organ of the body and consists of two layers: the outer epidermis and the inner dermis. The epidermis is the outer layer and protects the dermis. The epidermis can be subdivided into five layers.

The skin protects us from the environment, prevents the body from dehydrating, resists the invasion of micro organisms, protects against the harmful effects of ultraviolet light and assists in thermoregulation. Cells in the epidermis allow the surface of the skin to regenerate with the elastic and collagen fibres in the dermis making the skin tough and elastic.

In addition, you should have identified the four stages of the wound healing process:

(1) Vascular response or homeostasis
(2) Inflammation
(3) Proliferation
(4) Maturation

Included in your answer will have been a brief description of the four stages, that is, during the vascular response you will witness bleeding and the formation of a blood clot; the inflammatory stage protects from further damage; during proliferation lost tissue is replaced and collagen is formed to help strengthen the wound; finally, in the maturation stage, function and strength is restored, although the wound will never reach its pre-injury strength. You may also have identified the process of angiogenesis, where the formation of new capillaries is witnessed by the macrophages, thereby helping to oxygenate the wound.

REFERENCES

Barton, A. & Barton, A. (1981) *The Management and Prevention of Pressure Sores*. Faber & Faber, London.

Flanagan, M. (1997) *Wound Management*. Churchill Livingstone, New York.

Guyton, A. C. (1992) *Human Physiology and Mechanisms of Disease*. 5th edn. W. B. Saunders, Boston.

Morison, M. (2001) *The Prevention and Treatment of Pressure Ulcers*. Mosby, London.

Scales, J. T. (1990) Pathogenesis of pressure sores. In: *Pressure Sores Clinical Practice and Scientific Approach* (ed. Bader, D. L.), pp. 15–26. Macmillan Press, London.

Tortora, G. J. & Grabowski, S. R. (1999) *Principles of Anatomy and Physiology*. 9th edn. Harper Collins, New York.

Vannini, V. & Pogliani, G. (1999) *The New Atlas of the Human Body*. Chancellor Press, London.

Winter, G. D. (1962) Formation of the scab and the rate of epithelialisation of superficial wounds in the skin of the young domestic pig. *Nature*, **193**, 293–4.

Woolf, N. (1998) *Pathology: Basic and Systemic*. W. B. Saunders, London.

www.caretechlabs.com accessed 28 November 2003.

3 Aetiology of Pressure Ulcers and Principles of Pressure Ulcer Prevention

INTRODUCTION

This chapter will identify and discuss the aetiology of pressure ulcers, principles of pressure ulcer prevention, causes of pressure ulcers and the factors you need to consider when assessing and caring for your patient. Pressure, shear and friction are the true causes of pressure ulcer development but you must be aware of the other factors that may also determine an individual's susceptibility to their development. These concepts will be discussed within this chapter.

LEARNING OBJECTIVES

By the end of this chapter the reader will be enabled to:

❏ Discuss the aetiology of pressure ulcers
❏ Identify causes of pressure ulcers
❏ Discuss the causes of pressure ulcers
❏ Discuss principles of pressure ulcer prevention
❏ Identify intrinsic and extrinsic factors in the development of pressure ulcers

Aetiology of pressure ulcers

Pressure ulcers result from areas of previously healthy tissue becoming devitalised, resulting in localised skin death. Alexander *et al.* (2003) identify three examples where pressure ulcers may develop:

- As a result of direct, unrelieved pressure of soft tissues against bone
- Where friction occurs between the patient and the surface of a bed or chair
- As a result of shear force that frequently accompanies direct pressure and friction

The nature of the excessive pressure is important in the development of pressure ulcers. The principal factor in pressure ulcer development is excessive tissue pressure that prevents the normal supply of blood to the affected area. The normal mean capillary blood pressure is between 12 and 32 mmHg; therefore, pressure in excess of 30 mmHg will render tissue ischaemic and liable to damage and death (Burman, 1993). Indeed, lying on a hard floor generates surface interface pressures of 240 mmHg on the sacrum. A hospital mattress produces a standard interface pressure of between 21 and 71 mmHg (Agate, 1985). You can, therefore, see from these pressures, why many patients who have been found lying on a floor for a long period of time prior to admission, develop a pressure ulcer in the first few days following their admission. The severity of skin and tissue damage will depend on how long the patient has been exposed to these excess pressures.

It is worth noting here that many studies (Bennett & Lee, 1985; Bader & Grant, 1988; Schubert & Fagrell, 1991) have found that there are variations in the critical closing pressures in different patients. There is evidence that some patients are unable to respond to repetitive pressure loading of the skin even at comparatively low external pressures (Morison, 2001). Bader (1990) exposed both normal and debilitated patients to repetitive pressure of 30 mmHg and reported that some debilitated patients showed no recovery during the initial load application. Following load removal recovery was not fully achieved and subsequent loading had a cumulative effect on reducing transcutaneous oxygen. The same cumulative reduction in transcutaneous oxygen was observed for some debilitated patients positioned on a dynamic cushion support.

Dinsdale (1973) and Reswick and Rogers (1976) maintain that prolonged low pressure is as hazardous as short-term high pressure. Their studies examined the relationship between pressure and time, and ulcer and no ulcer. They reported an inverse relationship between the amount and duration of pressure, that is, low pressure for short periods caused ulceration. This clearly highlights the importance of regularly moving your patient's position; you must move your patients at regular intervals even if you are nursing them on a pressure redistributing device.

Braden and Bergstrom (1987) identified the term 'tissue tolerance' to explain the ability of the skin and its supporting structures to endure the effects of pressure without adverse affect. They distinguished between extrinsic and intrinsic factors affecting tissue tolerance.

The next section will identify and discuss the causes of pressure ulcers and the issues of extrinsic and intrinsic factors.

Causes of pressure ulcers

To be able to effectively prevent the development of a pressure ulcer the practitioner must understand the causes. Pressure damage may be referred to as a 'bed sore', 'pressure sore', 'decubitus ulcer' or 'pressure ulcer'. All these terms refer to the same problem encountered by many patients, and all are caused by the same common denominator: that of sustained pressure causing ischaemia (Farley, 2002). Technically, the term 'decubitus ulcer' refers to wounds developed over bony prominences while in the recumbent position, that is, sacrum, heel, or occiput, since *decumbere* means 'to lie down' in Latin. This would mean that wounds acquired from extended pressure in the seated position, that is, ischial, are not decubitus ulcers. In general, wounds acquired from pressure over bony prominences may always be referred to as pressure ulcers. The European Ulcer Advisory Panel (EPUAP, 1999) has defined a pressure ulcer as: 'an area of localised damage to the skin and underlying tissue caused by pressure, shear or friction or a combination of these'.

Pressure

Pressure can be described as a force exerted perpendicularly to the tissue, while shear is a force exerted parallel to the tissue. The combination of shear and pressure appears to be particularly damaging to the skin. Figures 3.1 and 3.2 identify the pressure points in lying and sitting positions. If a sufficient shearing force is present, only half the pressure is required to obtain vascular occlusion, compared with a situation without the presence of shearing. A pressure higher than the capillary pressure slows down the flow in the capillaries and lymph nodes, resulting in an insufficient supply of oxygen and nutrients and insufficient evacuation of metabolic waste (Defloor, 1999).

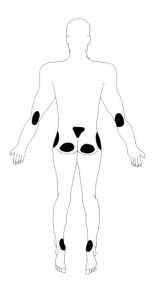

Fig. 3.1 Figure of potential pressure points in lying position.

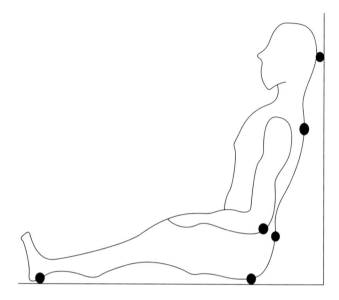

Fig. 3.2 Figure of potential pressure points in sitting position.

Friction

Friction occurs when the skin and another surface rub together. The other surface may include the cushion of a chair, bed sheets or incontinence sheets. Friction increases the probability of pressure ulcer development when accompanied by pressure and/or shearing forces. Friction can result in superficial damage through the stripping of the epidermis and may be exacerbated by the presence of moisture (Dealey, 1997; Defloor, 1999). Damage by friction is painful, as the nerve endings become exposed to the air. Dry skin also increases the risk of injury since elasticity is decreased (AHCPR, 1992). It is important to remember that not all pressure ulcers are caused by lying or sitting in one position for a period of time but may be due to devices used to implement care. For example, oxygen tubing may rub against the side of the face or may damage tissue around the patient's face or ears, especially when they are laid on their side and unable to reposition themselves without assistance. Nasogastric tubing may also be a potential factor for damage, as are intravenous cannula and catheters that the patient may be inadvertently laid on. Do not forget that if the patient is unconscious they will be unable to complain of pain and it is your duty to ensure that no potential pressure area damage will occur from the equipment being used.

Shear

Shear occurs when tissues are wrenched in opposite directions, resulting in disruption or angulation of capillary blood vessels, which may result in ischaemia and cell death. Gebhardt (1995) argued that pressure is rarely applied uniformly and there is, therefore, a degree of tissue deformation that creates shear forces that may damage the blood vessels.

Shearing forces often occur in patients who are in the semi-recumbent position for long periods of time. You may witness this happening when the patient is continually slipping down the bed or out of the chair. In these cases the epidermis remains static but the underlying tissues are pushed forward, that is to say, the skeleton remains still but the skin moves. This movement causes stretching and deformation of the capillary blood vessels and tissue ischaemia occurs. Bader and Grant (1988) stated that shearing forces can cause full-thickness tissue damage and are a precipitating factor in the development of many sacral and heel pressure ulcers. Shear reduces the external pressure required to stop blood flow in the skin, and there is evidence that high levels of shear halve the occlusion pressure (Bennett *et al.*, 1979). They also demonstrated that pressure was the primary force responsible for occlusion, but that a shear force was an important secondary factor.

All these factors must be taken into account. The causes may be divided into the three areas of extrinsic, intrinsic and external factors.

Pressure ulcer prevention

Successful pressure ulcer prevention results from removing these causes. It is important that pressure is relieved, particularly from over a bony prominence. Pressure damage usually occurs in the first few days following an acute episode of illness or enforced immobility (Gebhardt, 1992). This may be due to a variety of factors, including heart failure, vasomotor failure, vasoconstriction due to shock, pain, low blood pressure and temperature change, particularly during and after anaesthesia (Bliss, 1990; Scott, 2000). Indeed, an anaesthetised or semiconscious person has no independence to reposition him or herself. External pressure over the tissues will cause compression and distortion and if the pressure is significantly higher than the capillary closing pressure, generally stated as being 32 mmHg at the arteriolar end of the capillary bed and 12 mmHg at the venule end (Landis, 1930), then the result will be an occlusion of the blood vessels, potentially leading to ischaemia and cell death. Interestingly, Landis updated his work in 1941, and claims the accepted threshold should now be between 46 mmHg and 50 mmHg, with Bridel (1993) suggesting that the collagen content of the skin must also be considered. This is due to collagen acting as a buffer to external pressure and providing a degree of protection for the blood vessels.

The relevance of this becomes clear when considering the interface pressures recorded between major bony prominences of a patient and a standard NHS mattress. These have been reported as between 70 and 100 mmHg, thus exceeding capillary closing pressure (Collier, 1996).

It should be remembered that not everyone who lies on a hard surface which exerts a high pressure develops a pressure ulcer. Normally, an individual would move their own position when experiencing discomfort or pain. A susceptible individual may develop a pressure ulcer for a variety of reasons, for example, enforced bed rest, loss of sensation. Damage may result from high pressures over a short period of time or from lower pressures over a longer period of time. Bridel (1993) argues that once the critical values for pressure and time have been reached, tissue damage will proceed at a similar rate regardless of the degree of pressure being exerted.

Extrinsic factors

These factors are presented in box 3.1.

Box 3.1 Extrinsic factors.

The three factors in this area may be defined as:

- Pressure: the force applied vertically to a surface
- Shear: the force that is applied tangentially or in parallel (Bliss, 1993)
- Friction: resistance met by the body moving over another surface

---

Shearing forces may occur when an individual slides down the bed or chair. Inappropriate moving and handling techniques employed by practitioners may also result in shearing forces being exerted. Friction is the third factor that may result in damaged tissues. Defloor (1999) states that friction occurs when two surfaces move across each other. It often removes superficial layers of skin, with friction damage often occurring as a result of poor moving and handling techniques. In addition to the extrinsic factors there are the intrinsic factors.

Intrinsic factors

The intrinsic factors are presented in box 3.2.

Box 3.2 Intrinsic factors.

- Age
- Medications
- Low blood pressure
- Low skin temperature and raised body temperature
- Reduced mobility
- Chronic illness or disability
- Acute illness
- Poor oxygen perfusion in the tissues
- Poor nutrition
- Incontinence
- Emaciation/obesity
- Neurological deficit

A number of studies have suggested that advancing age is a significant intrinsic factor with pressure ulcer development. It has been demonstrated that the total collagen content of the skin falls at a steady rate between the ages of 30–80 years, with a gradual reduction in the synthesis of collagen from the ages of 20–60 years, followed by a dramatic fall in its synthesis over the age of 60 years. The administration of steroids also mimics the ageing process and leads to a reduction of collagen; however, this is reversible when the treatment is discontinued (Hall *et al.* 1981). In addition, the use of other medications may also put the patient at risk of developing pressure ulcers. For example, the use of diuretics may cause dehydration; sedatives may reduce natural sleep movement; cimetidine and ranitidine are associated with protein malabsorption and aspirin and anti-inflammatory medications are associated with iron deficiency anaemia. Therefore, it is important that your assessment of the patient includes a history of the medication they are currently prescribed and any past medications. It may also be worthwhile to ask relatives or carers to bring the patient's medication into hospital for you to check if they have not brought it with them on admission. Sometimes patients cannot remember exactly which type of medication they are prescribed and it is important that you document this information correctly.

Low systolic blood pressure has been found to be a factor in pressure ulcer development, with those patients who had a low systolic reading being found to be more at risk, due to an impaired reactive hyperaemia response. However, Cullum and Clark (1992) and Allman *et al.* (1995) found systolic and diastolic blood pressure readings to be non-significant in the development of pressure ulcers. We must also take into account that neonates and very young children are at risk of developing pressure ulceration. Their skin is still maturing and their head-to-body weight is disproportionate. Heath (2002) states that neonates have very fragile skin which can easily break down if they are not repositioned regularly. Tape stronger than micropore should not be used because the adhesive may tear the skin. Children who are malnourished, unconscious or immobilised in one area for any long period of time should be assessed for their risk of developing a pressure ulcer. Some of the sites that may be at a potential risk of pressure damage may differ from those of an adult, that is, on the ears from oxygen therapy, or from repeated heel pricks for blood tests.

People with learning disabilities who are confined to bed may have a higher risk of pressure ulcer development due to heavy sedation, or a lack of motivation to move independently. There are sometimes misconceptions regarding the amount of care a person with learning disabilities requires, for example, the failure to recognise basic needs such as assistance with feeding, hygiene, the ability to comprehend instructions or to communicate physical discomfort (Heath, 2002). You therefore need to be aware that this patient group will require assessment and health education regarding the prevention of pressure ulcer development.

General patient assessment

Skin inspection

Skin inspection must form a basis for your assessment of the patient; this should occur on an individual basis for each patient and the frequency should be determined in response to changes in the individual's condition and in relation to either deterioration or recovery (NICE, 2003). Please refer to Appendix Two for further information. The NICE guidelines recommend that skin inspection should be based on an assessment of the most vulnerable areas of risk for each patient. These include the heels; trochanters; ischial tuberosities; parts of the body affected by the wearing of anti-embolic stockings and parts of the body where pressure, shear and friction are exerted in the course of an individual's daily living activities. You should also inspect those areas that are affected by external forces exerted by equipment and clothing. This may include, the elbows, shoulders, back of the skull and toes.

When assessing the skin you will need to record any signs of persistent erythema; non-blanching hyperaemia; blisters; discolouration; localised heat; localised oedema and localised induration. In those patients who have darkly pigmented skin you will need to be assessing for any signs of purplish/bluish localised areas of skin; localised heat that, if tissue becomes damaged, is replaced by coolness; localised oedema and localised induration (NICE, 2003, 1.1.4.5).

Furthermore, the NICE guidelines continue to recommend that individuals who are willing should be encouraged to inspect their own skin following education. Those who use wheelchairs should use a mirror to inspect those areas not easily seen or ask someone else to inspect their skin. You must remember to ensure that when you are inspecting the patient's skin that you are aware of any predisposing medical conditions that may have an effect on the skin. These may include dermatology conditions or medications, such as steroids, that will make the skin vulnerable to damage.

Mobility

Reduced mobility is a major factor in pressure ulcer development. An immobile patient is unable to move their own position or weight sufficiently enough to relieve pressure. Intervention is, therefore, essential by the nurse or carer, who can aid in maintaining and enhancing functional ability. Referrals should also be made to the physiotherapist and occupational therapist to allow the formulation and implementation of an exercise regime. Remember, medical permission must be sought and obtained prior to undertaking any exercise with the immobile patient. Repositioning of the immobile patient is vitally important; the frequency should be based upon individual assessment and not ritualistic practice. Repositioning should avoid the patient's vulnerable areas, but at the same time, consideration must be given to the condition of the individual, medical conditions, mealtimes, personal hygiene and physiotherapy regimes, with the plan of care reflecting these issues. Prior to any patient being repositioned, risk assessment should be carried out and the results documented: whenever the patient is repositioned it must also be documented. The entries must be dated, timed and signed by the practitioner. If a student nurse or unqualified member of staff documents the care, a qualified practitioner must countersign these entries.

Practitioners should assess each patient's mobility status when determining their potential risk of pressure ulcer development, for example, what is the reason for the patient's immobility (post-operative, sensory, neurological); does the patient's medical condition allow mobility; is the patient motivated to move? Whatever the reason for the immobility status of the patient, a repositioning regime must be implemented on an individual basis to aid in the prevention of pressure ulcer formation. Patients with loss of sensation can be vulnerable to localised pressure and preventative strategies to protect the skin must be implemented, which includes educating the patient, relatives and carers on suitable clothing, footwear and changing their position at regular intervals.

Repositioning

It is important to remember that a regime of two-hourly turns is *not* acceptable for every patient. The NICE guidelines (2003) have recommended that individuals who are 'at risk' of pressure ulcer development should be repositioned and the frequency of repositioning determined by the results of skin inspection and individual needs, not by a ritualistic practice. Repositioning should take into consideration relevant matters, such as the patient's general medical condition, their comfort, the overall plan of care and the support surface being used.

How often should you reposition a patient?
Individual needs must be assessed and a regime planned, as the condition dictates. The practice of two-hourly turning regimes stemmed from classic studies performed by Norton (1989), who concluded that patients who were immobile were prone to developing pressure ulcers. However, she did not state that the optimal frequency for repositioning patients was two-hourly. Knox *et al.* (1994) suggested that patients might benefit from being repositioned every one and a half hours, with the frequency changing if the skin colour changed within 90 minutes of immobility. Some patients showed skin colour changes after one hour, which suggests that some patients will require hourly repositioning. This shows us that assessment of patients who are at risk of pressure ulcer development must be assessed on an individual basis. The

ritualistic practice of two-hourly turning should not be used for every patient.

The 30° tilt
The 30° tilt may prove useful in repositioning the patient. With this technique the head of the bed is elevated to 30°, with the patient's hips and shoulders being laterally tilted to a 30° position, with pillows or foam wedges being utilised to maintain the position. There should be no pressure on the sacrum or trochanters with this method. Colin *et al.* (1996), found this technique did not impair oxygen supply to the skin; whereas there was an impairment of oxygen to the skin in the 90° laterally inclined individual.

Moving and handling techniques
All staff involved in the repositioning and moving and handling of any patient must have undergone the mandatory training programme for safe moving and handling techniques and should be proficient in using any manual handling device. If a manual handling device is used then any slings utilised must be removed from under the patient following completion of the procedure and the device returned to its correct storage space. There are some slings that are made from silk and are more delicate on the skin. Patients may sometimes be left sitting or lying on these where it would be difficult to remove a sling, particularly in the community. Please note that manual handling devices such as hoists are not to be used for transferring the patient from the bed area to the toilet or day room. They are designed for the transfer of the individual from bed to chair or chair to bed only. It should be normal and acceptable practice that slings for the hoists are disposable and for one patient use only, to prevent the risk of cross-infection. Some trusts use slings that are washable. If the equipment is not disposable then the equipment must be cleaned as per the manufacturer's instructions and the infection control policy.

Please check your individual workplace's policies for this information.

Nutrition

Eating and drinking in adequate amounts is essential to life and good health. However, when a patient is admitted to hospital they often do not eat and drink in adequate amounts for a variety of reasons, for example, fasting prior to an operation, nil by mouth status due to their condition, unconsciousness, pain, chronic illness, acute illness, polypharmacy, mental disorders, physical disability, alcoholism, or poverty. This results in suboptimal nutrition or malnutrition, when the dietary intake of the individual does not meet the metabolic requirements. Due to the effect on the body tissues of the lack of nutrients it would seem that providing adequate nutrition is an essential component in the prevention of pressure ulcer development, with numerous studies identifying that many hospital patients are malnourished (Lennard-Jones, 1992; McWirter & Pennington, 1994).

Cross-sectional studies have suggested that a low protein and energy intake, low body weight, low serum albumin and haemoglobin levels may be associated with the development of pressure ulcers. Gilmore *et al.* (1995) noted that poor nutritional status was a sign of hypoalbuminaemia, with a poor food intake being associated with pressure ulcers. Protein has been widely reported as being an important dietary element in relation to the prevention of pressure ulcer development; however, there have been reports that low protein levels in patients with a pressure ulcer may have been caused by protein leaking from the wound in the exudate. It is, therefore, unclear as to whether the low protein levels have been caused as a result of the ulcer, or the ulcer being caused by a low protein intake.

The link between pressure ulcer development and nutrition is not universally accepted. There are problems in analysing the evidence and research design because nutritional factors affect the aetiology and healing of pressure ulcers or other types of chronic wounds. Many clinical studies have been carried out using animals and therefore it may be difficult to relate the findings directly to human beings, as there are anatomical, functional and metabolic differences between the two. Kemp *et al.* (1990) studied 125 surgical patients and found no direct association between those who had developed a pressure ulcer and falling serum albumin levels. Finucane (1995) concluded that although some studies do show a positive link between low serum albumin levels and pressure ulcer development others do not. However, most people do consider that malnutrition can be a reversible risk factor that is associated with pressure ulcer development and, therefore, care and strategies must be implemented to prevent patients suffering with malnutrition.

Maintaining nutrition

All patients should be assessed on admission for their potential risk of malnutrition; this may be carried out using the trust's nutritional assessment documentation. You should remember that it is not just the frail older person who is at risk but also younger patients, those who are obese and those whose medical conditions have affected their swallowing reflex. The results of your initial assessment should be documented in the care plan and dates for future assessments recorded. A referral to the dietician may be necessary on admission or during the patient's hospital stay. On discharge home it may be necessary to advise the patient, relatives or carers on how to maintain a well balanced diet and follow-up appointments to see the dietician may also be necessary. Extra support may be offered to the patients and their families on discharge, in the form of meals on wheels, visits to a day hospital or support from social services to help with shopping and preparation of meals. It may be necessary to provide education to the patient and relatives/carers regarding the importance of maintaining a well balanced diet and which foods constitute this. This information should be given to the patient, carers and relatives in verbal and written form.

When assessing the patient's nutritional status you should also identify any causative factors which may have led to the poor nutritional status, for example, does the patient suffer with any medical conditions which may prevent them from preparing food (for example, rheumatoid arthritis or reduced mobility), or are they on certain drug therapies that may depress the appetite? Visual assessment of the patient will indicate if they have been suffering with weight loss, that is, do they have ill fitting dentures, are clothes and jewellery loose, is there poor oral hygiene and does the patient appear disinterested when you ask them about their normal diet?

During the assessment process you should try and ascertain the dietary history of the patient. This will provide a baseline for the commencement of a dietary regime. Weighing the patient is important and should be carried out on admission and then weekly, if their admitting condition allows. If appropriate, the dietician will produce a nutritional care package for the patient; delivery of nutritional support will vary from patient to patient. If the gut is functional then oral feeding and the use of prescribed supplements may be indicated. If the gut is not functional then parental or enteral nutrition may be the treatment of choice.

The nurse should ensure that the patient receives and consumes the prescribed nutritional supplements as requested by the dietician. Meals should be presented attractively and help with feeding should be given as required. A dietary intake chart may need to be completed to assess and evaluate the levels of food and drink intake over a period of time. If this is necessary then all staff and relatives/carers must be aware that it is in progress and document all food and drink consumed by the patient. You should also take care that the patient and carers understand the reasons for the supplements and that discussions regarding the choice of oral supplements are undertaken with the patient to ensure that they receive supplements that are palatable to them. The patient's consent must be sought and documented prior to administering any nutritional support.

Remember that an interdisciplinary approach to maintaining the nutritional needs of the patient is required and, in addition to the nurse and dietician, medical staff may prescribe multivitamins and the speech therapist may be involved if the patient has swallowing difficulties. A variety of methods may be used to assess the nutritional status that include:

- Dietary history
- Physical examination
- Skin fold thickness
- Biochemical analysis, including plasma proteins, albumin levels, nitrogen balance and creatinine clearance and a full blood count

Parental nutrition may be administered following gut infarction, pancreatitis, gut resection, and cancers and trauma of the gut. Enteral nutrition is administered via nasogastric, gastrostomy or jejeunostomy tubes and may be required due to oropharyngeal obstruction, malabsorption, burns, chemotherapy, radiation therapy or neurological conditions. It is contraindicated in patients suffering with a paralytic ileus; intestinal obstruction beyond the duodenum; intractable vomiting, diarrhoea and gut bleeding; ischaemia; or severe inflammatory bowel disease.

Elimination

The patient who suffers with incontinence will require careful skin care. Constant washing and drying will result in a loss of skin elasticity; therefore the use of a skin cleanser and barrier cream will help to maintain moisture and protect the skin. Patients with diarrhoea may develop excoriation of the skin, so the use of incontinence products and a referral to the continence advisor may be beneficial, in addition to the patient being offered regular toileting. Skin should be inspected regularly for any signs of redness or excoriation, reported and documented, with action being implemented to prevent further deterioration.

All attempts must be made to maintain the patient's privacy and dignity, with the Department of Health (2001) recommending that patients should experience care in an environment that actively encompasses respect for their individual values, beliefs and personal relationships, and that the care promotes their privacy and dignity and protects their modesty.

Box 3.3 identifies the principles of pressure ulcer development.

Box 3.3 Principles of preventing pressure ulcer development.

- Assess individual for risk factors
- Ensure regular changes of position, assess each patient on an individual basis
- Maintain skin cleanliness and hygiene
- Prevent mechanical, physical and chemical injury
- Ensure adequate nutrition and hydration
- Promote control of continence
- Ensure good body alignment and positioning
- Use appropriate pressure redistributing systems
- Inspect the skin for any changes at regular intervals
- Promote mental alertness and orientation
- Educate all professionals and carers involved in the patient's skin care routine

Adapted from Walsh, M. (2002) *Watson's Clinical Nursing and Related Sciences*, 6th ed, p. 929, with kind permission from Elsevier Science Limited.

CONCLUSION

This chapter has discussed the various causes of pressure ulcers. We have seen that it is not just one factor that may cause the development of pressure ulcers but it may be a multitude of factors. It is, therefore, important that the patient is assessed in a holistic fashion rather than solely assessing their skin integrity. As a rule all patients, regardless of age or weight, should be assessed for the risk of developing a pressure ulcer on admission, and then reassessed as their condition dictates during their hospital stay, or if they are being nursed in the community, as their condition changes.

As well as taking the issues discussed in this chapter into account it may be necessary for you to choose a pressure re-distributing support system for your patient. Chapter six will describe the various systems available for you to choose from.

SELF-ASSESSMENT

After reading this chapter you should now take some time to reassess your knowledge base.

Reflection

Take some time to reflect upon the knowledge you have gained and how you will implement it into your own practice.

What knowledge did I possess prior to reading this chapter?

What do I know now?

How will my practice change as a result of attaining this knowledge?

Do I need to discuss with anyone practices I have witnessed that are not evidence-based, in relation to my new knowledge?

If so, who will I speak to?

Scenario

Complete this scenario based upon the knowledge you now possess.

Roger is a 49-year-old gentleman admitted to your ward with multiple sclerosis. He has been confined to a wheelchair for the past six months and he and his wife have been finding it increasingly difficult to maintain his skin integrity as his mobility has reduced greatly. On admission he presents with a purple area to his left and right heels, signs of excoriation on both his buttocks and a grade two ulcer to his left elbow, his right elbow is very red and painful to touch. He informs you that he has felt as if he is continually slipping out of his wheelchair and that he has been trying to prevent this by pushing up on his elbows and positioning his heels into the footplates of his wheelchair to stop him slipping down. In addition, he is suffering with urinary incontinence at night.

Tips on completing the scenario
Below is some information that you may have considered while working through the scenario. It is not an exhaustive list but it will give you some guidance on the information you should have collected.

You will need to revisit the use of risk assessment and grading tools. In addition, moving and handling and nutritional assessment tools will need to be examined. A holistic assessment of Roger will be required, identifying his activities of daily living and planning his care in line with these. As he already has skin damage you will need to plan a wound-dressing regime and support this with evidence, for example, the importance of maintaining a warm, moist healing environment (See Chapters Two and Seven).

Referrals to members of the interdisciplinary team will be necessary, for example, the physiotherapist and occupational therapist who can advise Roger and his wife on exercises for his muscles and chest and reassess his wheelchair and seating. It may also be necessary to refer him to a specialised wheelchair centre, as it would appear that his wheelchair no longer meets his needs (See Chapter 9).

The multiple sclerosis nurse specialist needs to be informed of his admission, as does the tissue viability specialist who will be able to advise on his wound care and pressure prevention strategy. His urinary incontinence at night will be distressing to both him and his wife and will be affecting his skin integrity; therefore, the specialist continence nurse will be required to offer advice. He may have a urinary tract infection, so a urine specimen should be obtained and sent to the laboratory for culture and sensitivity tests.

REFERENCES

Agate, J. (1985) Pressure sores. In: *Principles and Practice of Geriatric Medicine* (ed. Pathy, M.), Wiley, London.

Agency for Health Care Policy and Research (AHCPR) (1992) *Pressure Ulcers in Adults: Prediction and Prevention.* Clinical practice and guidelines, Number 3. Department of Health and Human Services. Md, US.

Alexander, M. F., Fawcett, J. N. & Runciman, P. J. (2003) *Nursing Practice: Hospital and Home.* Churchill Livingstone, Elsevier Science, London.

Allman, R. M., Goode, P. S., Patrick, M. N., Burst, N. & Bartolucci, A. A. (1995) Pressure ulcer risk factors among hospitalised patients with activity limitation. *Journal of American Medical Association*, **273** (11), 865–70.

Bader, D. L. & Grant, C. A. (1988) Changes in transcutaneous oxygen tension as a result of prolonged pressures at the sacrum. *Clinical Physiological Measurement*, **9**, 33–40.

Bader, D. (1990) *Pressure Sores: Clinical Practice and Scientific Approach.* Macmillan, London.

Bennett, L., Kavner, D., Lee, B. Y., Trainor, F. S. & Lewis, J. M. (1979) Shear versus pressure as causative factors in skin blood flow occlusion. *Archives of Physical Medicine and Rehabilitation*, **62** (8), 392–8.

Bennett, L. & Lee, B. Y. (1985) Pressure versus shear in pressure sore causation. In: *Chronic Ulcers of the Skin* (ed. Lee, B. Y.), Chapter Three. McGraw Hill, New York.

Bliss, M. (1990) Preventing pressure sores. (editorial). *Lancet*, **335**, 1311–2.

Bliss, M. (1993) Aetiology of pressure sores. *Clinical Gerontelogy*, **3**, 379–97.

Braden, B. & Bergstrom, N. (1987) A conceptual schema for the study of the aetiology of pressure sores. *Rehabilitation Nursing*, **12** (1), 8–16.

Bridel, J. (1993) The aetiology of pressure sores. *Journal of Wound Care*, **2** (4), 230–38.

Burman, P. (1993) Using pressure measurements to evaluate different technologies. *Decubitus*, **6** (3), 38–42.

Colin, D., Abraham, P. & Preault, L. (1996) Comparison of the 90 degree and 30 degree laterally inclined positions in the prevention of pressure ulcers using transcutaneous oxygen and carbon dioxide pressures. *Advances in Wound Care*, **9** (3), 35–8.

Collier, M. (1996) Pressure reducing mattresses. *Journal of Wound Care*, **5** (5), 207–11.

Collier, M. (2002) Caring for the patient with a skin or wound care need. In: *Watson's Clinical Nursing and Related Sciences* (ed. Walsh, M.), 6th edn. p. 929. Elsevier Science Limited, Edinburgh.

Cullum, N. & Clark, M. (1992) Intrinsic factors associated with pressure sores in elderly people. *Journal of Advanced Nursing*, **17** (4), 427–31.

Dealey, C. (1997) *Managing Pressure Sore Prevention*. Quay Books, Mark Allen Publishing Ltd, Salisbury.

Defloor, T. (1999) The risk of pressure sores: a conceptual scheme. *Journal of Clinical Nursing*, **8**, 206–16.

Department of Health (2001) *Essence of Care. Patient Focused Benchmarking for Health Care Practitioners*. Department of Health, London.

Dinsdale, S. M. (1973) Decubitus ulcers in swine: light and election microscopic study of pathogenesis. *Archives of Physical Medicine and Rehabilitation*, **55**, 147–52.

EPUAP European Ulcer Advisory Panel (1999) Guidelines on treatment of pressure ulcers. *Epuap Review*, **1**, 7–8.

Farley, M. (2002) Oh my, the pressure! *Operating Room Nursing Journal*, **20** (2), 9–13, 20.

Finucane, T. E. (1995) Malnutrition, tube feeding and pressure sores: data are incomplete. *Journal of American Geriatrics Society*, **43** (4), 447–51.

Gebhardt, K. (1992) Preventing pressure ulcers in orthopaedics. *Nursing Standard*, **6** (23), 9–13, 20.

Gebhardt, K. (1995) What causes pressure sores? *Journal of Wound Care*, **1** (4), 39–43.

Gilmore, S. A., Robinson, G., Posthauer, M. E. & Raymond, J. (1995) Clinical indicators associated with unintentional weight loss and pressure ulcers in elderly residents of nursing home facilities. *Journal of the American Dietetic Association*, **95**, 984–92.

Aetiology & Prevention of Pressure Ulcers | **3**

Hall, D. A., Blackett, A. D., Zajac, A. R., Switala, S. & Airey, C. M. (1981) Changes in skinfold thickness with increasing age. *Age and Ageing*, **10** (1), 19–23.

Heath, H. B. M. (2002) *Potter and Perry's Foundation in Nursing Theory and Practice.* Elsevier Science Limited, London.

Kemp, M. G., Keithley, J. K., Smith, D. W. & Morreale, B. (1990) Factors that contribute to pressure sores in surgical patients. *Research in Nursing and Health*, **13**, 293–301.

Knox, D. M., Anderson, T. M. & Anderson, P. S. (1994) Effects of different turn intervals on skin of healthy older adults. *Advances in Wound Care*, **7** (1), 48–52.

Landis, E. (1930) Microcirculation studies of capillary blood pressure in human skin. *Heart*, **15**, 209–28.

Lennard-Jones, J. E. (1992) *A Positive Approach to Nutrition as Treatment.* Kings Fund Centre for Health Services Development, London.

McWirter, J. P. & Pennington, C. (1994) Incidence and recognition of malnutrition in hospital. *British Medical Journal*, **308**, 945–8.

Morison, M. (2001) *The Prevention and Treatment of Pressure Ulcers.* Mosby, London.

National Institute for Clinical Excellence (2003) *Pressure Ulcer Prevention. Pressure Ulcer Risk Assessment and Prevention; Including the Use of Pressure-relieving Devices (Beds, Mattresses and Overlays) for the Prevention of Pressure Ulcers in Primary and Secondary Care.* NICE Clinical guideline No 7. National Institute for Clinical Excellence, London. Available from: www.nice.org.uk

Norton, D. (1989) Calculating the risk: reflections on the Norton Scale. *Decubitus* (August), 24–31.

Reswick, J. B. & Rogers, J. (1976) Experience at Ranchos Los Amigos Hospital with devices and techniques to prevent pressure sores. In: *Bedsore Biomechanics* (eds Kenedi, R. M., Cowden, J. M. & Scales, J. T.), pp. 301–11. Macmillan Press, London.

Schubert, V. & Fagrell, B. (1991) Post-occlusive reactive hyperaemia and thermal response in the skin microcirculation of subjects with spinal cord injury. *Scandinavian Journal of Rehabilitation Medicine*, **23** (1), 33–40.

Scott, E. M. (2000) The prevention of pressure ulcers in the operating department. *Journal of Wound Care*, **8** (9), 437–41.

Walsh, M. (2002) *Watson's Clinical Nursing and Related Sciences*, 6th edn. Elsevier Science Limited, Edinburgh.

Risk Assessment

4

This chapter will discuss the importance of accurate risk assessment, how to identify an individual at risk of developing a pressure ulcer and provide several examples of risk assessment tools that you may witness in the clinical areas. You will find it useful to refer to Appendices Two and Three throughout this chapter.

LEARNING OBJECTIVES

By the end of this chapter the reader will be enabled to:

❏ Identify risk assessment tools
❏ Discuss the use of these tools
❏ Identify individuals 'at risk' of developing a pressure ulcer
❏ Identify and discuss guidelines relevant to identifying individuals at risk

INTRODUCTION

A crucial feature for the prevention of pressure ulcers is correct and early identification of patients at risk. You may find it useful to use a risk assessment tool to help you identify certain individuals, but remember that these tools are not designed to replace clinical judgement, but are part of a holistic assessment. The majority of patients admitted to a care setting, including those patients who are being nursed in a community setting, should be assessed, regardless of their age, gender or weight, and the results documented. Each patient will then be given a date for reassessment. However, it may not be appropriate for those patients admitted to an acute mental health unit (patients admitted to an elderly mental health unit should be assessed), obstetrics or paediatrics. If a patient is assessed as being at risk, then preventative measures should be implemented immediately and documented. Failure to do so may be viewed as a negligent act on the part of the practitioner, as the patient may develop skin damage, which will be seen as harming the patient and may be viewed as a breach of human rights, as discussed in Chapter One.

Identifying individuals 'at risk'

All individuals admitted to hospital or within a community setting should have an 'at risk' assessment performed within six hours of their initial admission (NICE, 2003). However, some hospitals and community settings state that assessment must be carried out within two hours of admission and reassessment must take place weekly, or more often if there is a sudden change in the patient's condition. You must, therefore, refer to your own local guidelines for the relevant policy for this assessment.

Please refer to Appendix Two for further information on the NICE guidelines regarding pressure ulcer prevention. If the patient is considered to be 'not at risk' then reassessment should be performed if, and when, their condition changes. If the patient is assessed to be 'at risk' then an immediate preventative plan of care must be implemented. The risk assessment should be performed by an appropriately trained member of staff who possesses the required knowledge, expertise and training to carry out the assessment and who is able to recognise the risk factors that may contribute to the development of pressure ulcers. They should be able to initiate effective preventative measures or, indeed, measures to treat established pressure ulcers if appropriate. This is supported by the NICE guidelines (2003).

Who should undertake the assessment?

As a rule it will tend to be a member of the nursing staff who will carry out the initial assessment. However, it is acceptable for medical staff, therapists or carers to carry out the assessment if they have had the appropriate training. Remember that your results must be documented immediately following the assessment and made available to all members of the interdisciplinary team. The Department of Health (2001, factors 1, 2, 3, 4, 8 and 9) state that the individualised plans of care should be agreed in partnership with the patient, relatives, carers and members of the interdisciplinary team. They do not promote developing a plan of care without the involvement of these people. Please refer to Appendix Three for further information relating to the *Essence of Care* guidelines for pressure ulcers.

When to reassess

Reassessment dates should be calculated on an individual basis, so this may be daily or weekly, but must be carried out more frequently if the patient's condition changes at any time. You will need to find out which risk assessment tool your trust utilises and make yourself familiar with it. If you are uncertain how to complete the documentation, ask for advice from relevantly trained qualified nurses and/or the tissue viability specialist.

NICE (2003) states that an individual's potential to develop pressure ulcers may be influenced by a variety of factors that all require consideration by the practitioner undertaking a patient assessment. These factors can be seen in Box 4.1.

Your initial skin assessment of the patient will identify if they are 'at risk', or not 'at risk', or if they already have an established pressure ulcer. The treatment to be prescribed will be derived from this information. Remember, if the patient has a pressure ulcer then you will need to implement not only preventative measures but also measures to treat the pressure ulcer. The Department of Health (2001) states that patients at

---

Box 4.1 Risk factors.

- Pressure
- Shear
- Friction
- Reduced mobility or immobility
- Sensory impairment
- Acute illness
- Level of consciousness
- Extremes of age
- Vascular disease
- Severe chronic or terminal illness
- Previous history of pressure damage
- Malnutrition and dehydration

Adapted with kind permission from the National Institute for Clinical Excellence (2003) *Pressure Ulcer Prevention. Pressure Ulcer Risk Assessment and Prevention; including the use of Pressure-relieving Devices (Beds, Mattresses and Overlays) for the Prevention of Pressure Ulcers in Primary and Secondary Care.* NICE Clinical Guideline No 7. National Institute for Clinical Excellence, London. Available from: www.nice.org.uk

---

risk of developing pressure ulcers should be cared for on a pressure redistributing support surface that meets their individual needs, including comfort (refer to Chapter Six).

National Institute of Clinical Excellence (NICE) Guidelines

The NICE guidelines relating to pressure ulcer prevention are Clinical Guideline 7 (NICE, 2003) and have been produced to provide a coordinated approach to risk assessment and prevention of pressure ulcers. The guidelines encompass pressure ulcer risk assessment, including the use of pressure-relieving devices (beds, mattresses and overlays), for the prevention of pressure ulcers in primary and secondary care (NICE, 2003). They state that all members of the interdisciplinary team should be aware of the guidelines, and all care administered should be documented in the patient's healthcare records. This means that the guidelines are intended to be used by all healthcare staff, including managers, professionals allied to medicine, nurses, doctors, equipment suppliers and academics. They may also be adopted for use by patients and carers.

You should make yourself familiar with these guidelines but note that all its recommendations may not be appropriate for use in all clinical settings and, therefore, you must also use your own professional judgement.

The following list requires consideration when undertaking an assessment:

- Available resources and equipment
- Local services, policies and protocols
- Individual patient needs
- Clinical experience of the practitioner
- The most up-to-date research and evidence

These guidelines were first produced in spring 2000 and revision took place in 2003. Review of the guidelines is expected again in four years time with updated guidelines being available within two years of the start of the review process.

Risk assessment tools

There are numerous risk assessment tools that have been developed and implemented over the years but they only act as an aide-memoire and should never replace clinical judgement. These tools will assist in raising your awareness of the risk factors, provide a minimum standard of risk assessment, provide a prompt for risk assessment, improve documentation, provide a crude indicator of risk and provide a framework for care provision. They will not distinguish between an actual pressure ulcer, potential problems of skin changes or a potential 'at risk' problem, neither will they distinguish between pressure factors or skin tolerance factors. They are a snapshot view of the patient's condition at a given point in time and do not predict differing skin responses or patient circumstances (Morison, 2001).

Different risk assessment tools include a range of risk factors. However, there is little research evidence to support the decisions reached for each tool but practitioners do support the choices made. What should be noted when you choose your system, is that it has been designed for the patient group you are caring for and that you have received the education and support to use the tool effectively. For example, the Walsall tool (Milward *et al.* 1993), was designed for use specifically in a community setting. If it were to be used in a hospital setting then you would experience over or under prediction of the 'at risk' status of the patient.

Using an 'at risk' tool
Before you use a risk assessment tool, ensure that you are familiar with its components. If you are unfamiliar, then spend some time researching the tool. Ask the tissue viability link specialist on your unit to show you how to use it and to explain why this tool has been selected for use on your ward or unit. Reassess your patient at regular intervals and ensure that the new assessment is documented alongside the new date for reassessment, with the rationale for the documented care. All staff on the ward or unit should be familiar with the tool and if there are teaching sessions for its use or new innovations in assessing patients at risk then try to attend them. This will allow you to keep updated and will offer you the opportunity to ask questions. When you attend these sessions do not forget to reflect on the activity and record it in your personal portfolio.

The following are examples of risk assessment tools you may see in clinical areas:

- **Braden**
  This tool is composed of six categories: sensory perception, moisture, activity, mobility, nutrition, and friction and shear. Numerical values are assigned to each category, which then gives the patient their 'at risk' score. A score of 16 or below

is claimed to be indicative that a patient is at risk of developing a pressure ulcer; the range of scores is between 6 and 23. The lower the score the higher the risk; therefore 6 indicates high risk. This tool is widely used in the USA but is less popular in the UK. However, you may well witness its use in some healthcare environments.

- **Douglas**

  This tool is aimed at general medical ward patients and is composed of seven categories: nutritional state/haemoglobin, activity, incontinence, pain, skin state, mental state, and special risk factors, including diabetes and steroid therapy. Each category is assigned a numerical value, with the lower the score the greater the risk of the patient developing a pressure sore. The highest score is 23, indicating low risk, the lowest score is 6, indicating high risk.

- **Knoll**

  This tool is aimed at acute care patients and is composed of eight categories: general state of health, mental status, activity, mobility, incontinence, oral nutritional intake, oral fluid intake and predisposing diseases (diabetes, neuropathies, vascular disease, anaemia). Numerical values are assigned to each category, with the higher the score the greater the risk. The highest score is 33; scores above 12 indicate that the patient is at risk.

- **Norton**

  This tool was developed following observations of elderly patients by Norton *et al.* (1962). She collected data that suggested the important characteristics in terms of the development of pressure ulcers. These included: general physical condition, mental state, activity, mobility and incontinence. She used these points to develop her tool, with each category being given a score of between one and four. A low score indicates that the patient is at high risk of developing a pressure ulcer; whereas a high score indicates that the patient's likelihood of developing a pressure ulcer is low. Generally a score of 14 is considered to be the risk threshold. The scale does not take into account the nutritional status of the patient, aetiological factors or patients who are to undergo surgery and, as such, has received much criticism. This scale is no longer widely used but you may well find it within care of the older adult environments.

- **Pressure Sore Prediction Scale**

  This tool is aimed at orthopaedic patients and composed of six categories. These include: sitting up, unconscious, poor general condition, incontinence and mobility. Each category is assigned a numerical value and the higher the score the more at risk the patient is perceived to be. The highest score is 16 indicating high risk, with a score of 6 or above being at risk.

- **Waterlow**

  Judy Waterlow developed this tool to help nurses who were working within medical or surgical units. Her aims were to provide guidelines on the selection of preventative aids and equipment, and management of established pressure ulcers. She stated that these would promote the user's awareness of the causes of pressure ulcers, thus promoting a means of determining the risk of pressure ulcer development. She included nutrition, tissue malnutrition, neurological deficit, surgery/trauma and medication as risk sections.

  Again, as with the other scales, the patient is assigned a numerical value for each category. The higher the numerical value the more 'at risk' the patient is perceived to be of developing pressure ulcers. The risk threshold is deemed to be 10, but there are varying degrees of risk above this number, that is:

10–15	at risk
15–20	high risk
20 and above	very high risk.

There would appear to be very little, if any, actual research or scientific evidence behind the development of this scale but it does remain popular and is used by many healthcare providers.

- **Medley**

  This tool was developed with an array of various categories. As with the Waterlow Scale it encompasses nutrition, predisposing disease, skin condition, incontinence, activity, mobility, pain and level of consciousness. The patient is assigned a numerical value for each category, although more than one choice may be made in each category. The higher the numerical value the more at risk the patient is perceived to be. The patients are split into three risk groups:

Low risk	0–9
Medium risk	10–19
High risk	20–36

- **Anderson**

  This was developed in Denmark for patients admitted with acute conditions and for use by non-medical personnel. The scale is split into two risk criteria; an absolute score that scores a point of two and include unconsciousness, dehydration and paralysis. The second criterion is that of a relative score, which scores a point of one, and includes age, mobility, incontinence, emaciation and redness over bony prominences. More than one choice can be made from each category; however, there is no division into degrees of risk, any single one factor on the absolute column puts the patients at risk.

Table 4.1 gives a review of the risk assessment tools we have discussed in this chapter.

Table 4.1 Review of risk assessment tools.

Risk assessment tool	Brief overview of tool
Braden	Six assessment categories. The LOWER the score the higher the predicted risk.
Douglas	Seven assessment categories. The LOWER the score the higher the predicted risk. Developed for use with general medical ward patients.
Knoll	Eight assessment categories. The HIGHER the score the higher the predicted risk. Developed for acutely ill patients.
Norton	Five assessment categories. The LOWER the score the higher the predicted risk. Developed for use with the older adult. No longer widely used, as it does not take nutrition into account.
Pressure Sore Prediction	Six assessment categories. The HIGHER the score the higher the predicted risk. Developed for orthopaedic patients.
Waterlow	Eleven assessment categories. The HIGHER the score the higher the predicted risk.
Medley	Eight assessment categories. The HIGHER the score the higher the predicted risk.
Anderson	Eight assessment categories. The HIGHER the score the higher the predicted risk. More than one choice may be made from each category. Developed for patients with acute conditions.

How valid are these tools?

When using these tools it is interesting to note that McGough (1999) carried out a systematic review of 43 risk assessment tools and found that only six had been tested for their predictive validity. Of the six, the Braden scale had been subjected to the greatest testing across community and hospital settings. However, other researchers have been unable to replicate these findings, so you should be cautious of relying too heavily upon the results of the risk assessment tools.

The *Effective Health Care Bulletin* (1995) suggests that there is no evidence that risk assessment scales are better than nurses' judgement in identifying patients at risk and that there is, in fact, no evidence to determine whether risk assessment scales are effective in reducing the incidence of pressure ulcers. Nevertheless, it is important that you adhere to policies of your own place of work in respect to the use of these risk assessment scales.

CONCLUSION

In conclusion, the risk assessment scales have been developed in an attempt to provide a structure and consistency in patient assessment, and as Watts and Clark (1993) determined, in a review of 138 pressure ulcer prevention policies, 90% of clinical areas recommended their use, which would suggest that nurses value them. They probably encourage nurses to maintain their knowledge base in this area and ensure that skin care protocols are developed for the clinical areas. Whichever tool you decide to use, it will provide a framework to work to and allow you to develop the patient's care in an individualised manner.

SELF-ASSESSMENT

After reading this chapter you should now take some time to reassess your knowledge base.

Reflection

Take some time to reflect upon the knowledge you have gained and how you will implement it into your own practice.

What knowledge did I possess prior to reading this chapter?

What do I know now?

How will my practice change as a result of attaining this knowledge?

Do I need to discuss with anyone practices I have witnessed that are not evidence-based, in relation to my new knowledge?

If so, who will I speak to?

Scenario

Complete this scenario based upon the knowledge you now possess.

The risk assessment tool currently being used on your ward is being re-evaluated. You are a newly qualified staff nurse on a care of the older person unit who has expressed an interest in becoming the associate tissue viability link nurse for your ward. The ward manager has asked you to participate with the link nurses in managing this re-evaluation and the subsequent changes that may be required.

Tips on completing the scenario
Below is some information that you may have considered while working through the scenario. It is not an exhaustive list but it will give you some guidance on the information you should have collected.

You will need to identify and investigate the various risk assessment tools available and examine the evidence for their use, with particular emphasis on the needs of the older person, for example, nutrition, predisposing diseases, skin condition, mental status and weight.

You will also need to access and read relevant national and local guidelines, policies and procedures relevant to the use of risk assessment tools. These will include the NICE guidelines and information published in the *Effective Care Bulletins*.

> **Further areas for investigation**
> Change management, leadership and motivation theories.
> These issues will help you to understand the principles of
> change management and how you would implement a new
> idea into a clinical area. Examples of these include work by
> Lewin and Adair.

REFERENCES

Adair, J. (1988) *The Action-centred Leader*. Biddles Ltd, Guildford, King's Lynn.

Department of Health (2001) *Essence of Care. Patient Focused Benchmarking for Health Care Practitioners*. Department of Health, London.

Effective Health Care Bulletin (1995) The prevention and treatment of pressure sores: how effective are pressure-relieving interventions and risk assessment for the prevention and treatment of pressure sores? *Effective Health Care Bulletin*, **1** (8), 1–11.

Lewin, K. (1951) *Field Theory in Social Science*. Harper and Row, New York.

A. J. McGough, 'A Systematic Review of the Effectiveness of Risk Assessment Scales used in the Prevention and Management of Pressure Sores', M.Sc. thesis (University of York, 1999).

Milward, P., Poole, M. & Skitt, T. (1993) Tissue viability. Pressure sore prevention: scoring pressure sore risk in the community. *Nursing Standard*, **7**, 50–5.

Morison, M. (2001) *The Prevention and Treatment of Pressure Ulcers*. Mosby, London.

National Institute for Clinical Excellence (2003) *Pressure Ulcer Prevention. Pressure Ulcer Risk Assessment and Prevention; including the use of Pressure-relieving Devices (Beds, Mattresses and Overlays) for the Prevention of Pressure Ulcers in Primary and Secondary Care*. NICE Clinical guideline No 7. National Institute for Clinical Excellence, London. Available from: www.nice.org.uk

Norton, D., McLaren, R. & Exton-Smith, A. N. (1962) *An Investigation of Geriatric Nursing Problems in Hospital*. National Corporation for the Care of Older People, London.

Royal College of Nursing (2001) *Pressure Ulcer Risk Assessment and Prevention Recommendations*. NICE Guidelines. Royal College of Nursing, London.

Watts, S. & Clark, M. (1993) *Pressure Sore Prevention: a Review of Policy Documents*. Nursing Practice Research Unit, University of Surrey, Guildford.

Grading Systems

5

INTRODUCTION

The purpose of this chapter is to introduce the reader to grading systems for all types of wounds, including pressure ulcers. Grading systems are those tools used to determine the severity of the established ulcer. Many systems exist to measure this and it is up to you to seek out which systems are being used in your place of work. If you are unfamiliar with the system you must ask for help and advice to guide you on how to use them accurately. Please note that these are only tools to assist you and are not a substitute for clinical judgement.

LEARNING OBJECTIVES

By the end of this chapter the reader will be enabled to:

❏ Identify various grading systems
❏ Discuss why a grading system may be used
❏ Identify signs that may indicate pressure
❏ Discuss what information should be documented when assessing a wound

Why use grading system?

A grading system assists in assessing the severity of the ulcer and gives a baseline onto which you can plan your care. Each grading system is divided into stages of pressure ulcer or wound severity. Some authors suggest that stage one or stage two skin damage is caused by pressure that is exerted parallel to the skin, caused by friction or shear damage on the skin surface. Stage three ulcers extend into the subcutaneous tissue but not through the fascia; whereas stage four ulcers are the deepest and involve the muscles, tendons and ligaments. Some form of pressure that leads to ischaemia causes all the ulcers. Stage one and two ulcers are classed as partial thickness as they do not extend beyond the epidermis and dermis. The majority of the healing occurs with regeneration of the epithelium. The new epithelium comes around the wound edges and is moist, allowing cells to migrate, to speed up the healing process. Stage three and four ulcers are full thickness, with both the epidermis and dermis being affected. Healing occurs through the development of new granulation tissue, epithelialisation and contraction.

During the granulation stage, new capillaries are formed and collagen is laid down. This gives the wound a red colour and should not be confused with inflammation or infection. Granulation normally occurs from the bottom of the wound upwards and, therefore, the depth of the wound will decrease as this stage develops. During epithelialisation the epithelial cells begin to surround and cover the wound across its base and sides. You may find it useful to revisit Chapter Two to refresh yourself on the anatomy and physiology of the skin and wound-healing process.

Grading systems

If all practitioners were using the same system then logic would dictate that all ulcers would be assessed objectively. However, this is not always the case and many of the systems available can be rather subjective, with different practitioners attributing various interpretations to the assessment. They do, though, help to provide a baseline for everyone to work with. The grading systems also assist in the incidence and prevalence studies that are undertaken. They provide information on the number of pressure ulcers in a specific care environment to the auditors undertaking the prevalence and incidence studies.

Prior to treating any pressure ulcer it is necessary first to grade it using a grading system. Several systems exist and it is vital that you document which one you are using and reassess it as necessary during the treatment of the ulcer. The following section will explain how to identify risk factors and how to accurately grade an ulcer.

Identification of risk factors

Understanding risk factors when assessing a patient with a pressure ulcer is vitally important, as it will allow you to be able to formulate an effective plan of care. If you are unsure as to how to use these tools then you must seek advice and education in their use. You should be aware of the following signs that may indicate initial pressure:

- Persistent erythema
- Non-blanching hyperaemia
- Blisters
- Discolouration
- Localised heat, oedema or induration
- Purplish-blue discolouration and localised heat in darkly pigmented skin

When you are grading a pressure ulcer the system is only a tool and you will also need to use your professional judgement in determining the severity of the ulcer. In addition take into account the patient's general condition, comfort, overall plan of care and the support surface that you may utilise or be utilising at the time of the assessment. It must be remembered that pressure ulcers must be assessed at regular intervals and not on a 'one-off' basis. The reassessment dates will be decided on an individual basis; therefore, each patient will have different reassessment dates.

The use of the grading systems offers the practitioner an indication of the progression of the ulcer and allows treatment to be evaluated and, if appropriate, changed. The NPUAP

(1989) recommends that ulcers be staged to describe the degree of injury and not to measure healing. Healing, they state, is measured using the wound size and characteristics of the wound.

Grades of ulcers

The EPUAP (1999) recognise that grade 1 pressure ulcers are difficult to measure in people with dark pigmented skin, and therefore have proposed a definition of grade 1 as being, non-blanchable erythema of intact skin, the heralding lesion of skin ulceration. In individuals with darker skin, warmth, oedema, induration, or hardness, may also be indicators. Grading a pressure ulcer will allow you to be able to determine the size, width, depth and severity of the ulcer.

The most common grading ranges are between 1 to 4 and 1 to 5. The differences between the numbers is due to the discussion over grade 1; some authors will identify a grade 1 ulcer as persistent blanching erythema, whereas others will classify it as being non-blanching erythema. The EPUAP (1999) recognise non-blanching erythema as grade 1. However, it is wise to remember that if an ulcer is covered by thick necrotic black eschar it will be impossible to accurately grade the ulcer and the degree of tissue damage until the eschar is removed. Therefore, it is recommended that you delay grading the ulcer until it is removed. You must document this decision in the patient's care plan with your rationale; for example, you may wish to document the size, site, colour and odour of the ulcer and then document that accurate grading cannot be performed at this time as the ulcer is covered by black eschar. The ulcer will be graded when the eschar has been removed. This will allow for the person who assesses it next, if it is not you, to understand why you have not graded the ulcer. It may also be that, when the eschar has been removed the ulcer actually appears to be larger in size. Do not panic, as this is due to the fact that the necrotic tissue may have masked the extent of tissue damage. When the necrotic tissue has been removed it will be replaced by slough, which is a combination of fibrous tissue and exudate. It is important that you remove both of these as soon as is possible, as both support infection. Removal may be by the use of appropriate dressings or by mechanical debridement. If mechanical debridement is to be used, this must be undertaken by an appropriately trained competent person and not undertaken by a student nurse.

During the assessment process you may notice that the ulcer appears to be travelling up and along the underside of the skin. This is known by a variety of terms, including *tunnelling*, *tracking* or *undermining*. If this is noted then it is important that the extent of the tunnelling is recorded, by probing the length of the ulcer with a suitable sterile instrument. This should not damage or extend the wound during the procedure. Again, a suitably trained professional, not a student nurse, must perform this procedure. When planning the treatment for this type of ulcer it is important that you promote healing from the distal aspect of the wound to prevent abscess formation in the future. Your observations must be recorded in the nursing care plan.

It is wise to remember that when you are using a grading system you are not only assessing the ulcer itself but also the surrounding skin. You will need to observe whether or not the surrounding skin appears red, macerated and hot to touch, or if there are any breaks in it. If there are then it may be indicative that the ulcer has spread and this will need to be recorded in the care plan. It is quite useful to compare it to the skin on the opposite side of the body.

The following section will discuss several grading systems, although others are available for use.

Examples of grading systems

The following examples of grading systems will serve as aide-memoire for you when assessing the ulcer.

Surrey system

This is one of the simplest tools to use, although you may have to be careful, as it may be quite subjective due to its simplicity. It employs four grading criteria as set out in the table 5.1. The EPUAP (1999) published their four grading system, which is similar to the Surrey system but contains more explanation for each grade. Table 5.2 illustrates this.

Table 5.1 Surrey system. Reproduced from Dealey, C. (1997) *Managing Pressure Sore Prevention.* Quay Books, Salisbury, with kind permission from Mark Allen Publishing Ltd.

Grade 1	Non-blanching erythema
Grade 2	Superficial break to the skin
Grade 3	Destruction of the skin without cavity
Grade 4	Destruction of the skin with cavity

Table 5.2 EPUAP grading system. Reproduced with kind permission from the European Pressure Ulcer Advisory Panel.

Grade 1	Non-blanchable erythema of intact skin; the heralding lesion of skin ulceration.
Grade II	Partial thickness skin loss involving epidermis and/or dermis. The ulcer is superficial and presents clinically as an abrasion, blister or shallow crater.
Grade III	Full thickness skin loss involving damage or necrosis of subcutaneous tissue that may extend down to, but not through underlying fascia. The ulcer presents clinically as a deep crater with or without undermining of adjoining tissue.
Grade IV	Full thickness skin loss with extensive destruction, tissue necrosis or damage to muscle, bone or supporting structures. Undermining and sinus tracts may be associated with stage IV pressure ulcers.

Stirling pressure sore severity scale

This scale (Reid & Morison, 1994) is another grading system that you may witness in practice. This also has four grades from 0–4, with grade 0 indicating no evidence of a pressure ulcer. The main difference of this system from the two already mentioned is that each grade has subsections, which are given a digit. The first two digits relate to the level and nature of tissue damage present, the third digit relates to the description of the wound bed and the fourth digit is a code for infection. This is a more detailed system than the others but may prove confusing to practitioners new to wound care. It requires practitioners to undertake training in how to use it effectively. Table 5.3 displays the Stirling Pressure Sore Severity Scale.

Torrance grading system

This tool was particularly popular in the 1990s and may still be seen in some care environments. However, it has lost popularity due to the fact that it is a five stage grading system. It was, though, relatively easy to use and is worth mentioning here for interest purposes. Table 5.4 below displays the Torrance grading system. Interestingly, with this grading system Torrance has made reference and provision for the possibility of infection.

None of the grading systems are one hundred per cent reliable and practitioners must be aware of this. Healey (1995) stated that the Torrance, Surrey and Stirling grading systems did not demonstrate any great level of reliability. However, the Stirling system was the least reliable as it had the most categories and nurses often did not accurately report their findings. Nonetheless, they do form a basis on which to base your plan of care and they ensure that each practitioner is following the same format in their assessment of the wound. Table 5.5 gives an overview of the grading systems we have discussed in this chapter.

As mentioned earlier, clinical judgement must always be used alongside these tools and advice sought where necessary.

NICE (2003) states that the risk assessment tools should only be used as an aide-memoire and should not replace clinical judgement. Please refer to Appendix Two for further information regarding the content of the NICE guidelines, clinical guideline 7.

Table 5.3 Stirling grading system. Reproduced from Phillips, J. (1997) *Access to Clinical Education. Pressure Sores*, p. 20, with kind permission from Elsevier Science Ltd.

Stage	Description
	No clinical evidence of a pressure ulcer
0.0	Normal appearance, intact skin
0.1	Healed with scarring
0.2	Tissue damaged but not assessed as a pressure ulcer
	Discolouration of intact skin
1.1	Non-blanchable erythema with increased local heat
1.2	Blue/purple/black discolouration
	Partial thickness skin loss involving epidermis and/or dermis
2.1	Blister
2.2	Abrasion
2.3	Shallow ulcer without undermining of adjacent tissue
2.4	Any of these with blue/purple/black discoloration or induration
	Full thickness skin loss involving damage or necrosis to subcutaneous tissue but not extending to underlying bone, tendon or joint capsule
3.1	Crater, without undermining of adjacent tissue
3.2	Crater, with undermining of adjacent tissue
3.3	Sinus, the full extent of which is uncertain
3.4	Full thickness skin loss, but wound bed is covered with necrotic tissue which masks the true extent of tissue damage
	Full thickness skin loss with extensive destruction and tissue necrosis extending to underlying bone, tendon, or joint capsule
4.1	Visible exposure of bone, tendon or capsule
4.2	Sinus assessed as extending to bone, tendon or capsule

Table 5.4 Torrance grading system. Reproduced from Phillips, J. (1997) *Access to Clinical Education. Pressure Sores*, p. 20, with kind permission from Elsevier Science Ltd.

Grade	Description
1	Blanching hyperaemia
2	Non-blanching hyperaemia
3	Ulceration progresses through the dermis only
4	The lesion extends into the subcutaneous fat
5	Infective necrosis penetrates the deep fascia

Table 5.5 Review of grading systems.

Grading system	Brief overview of content
Surrey system	Four stage grading criteria. Simple to use.
European Pressure Ulcer Advisory Panel (EPUAP) system	Four stage grading criteria. Contains detailed explanation for each stage. This tends to be the system of choice for healthcare professionals.
Stirling system	Four stage grading criteria, further subdivided to allow the person completing the assessment to: • Assess the level of tissue damage present • Describe the wound bed • Record any signs of infection
Torrance system	Five stage grading criteria. Provision is made for the possibility of infection.

Assessment of the ulcer

When assessing the wound you will need to document:

- Position of the ulcer
- Appearance
- Size
- Condition of surrounding skin
- Odour
- Exudate levels

- Any pain that the patient may have in relation to the wound and surrounding areas
- Any signs of clinical infection
- Assessment of the wound bed

These observations should be made at each dressing change and documented in the nursing care plans. Your documentation of the wound should include measurements of the diameters of the wound margins, which may be drawn, traced on acetate, or photographed, depending upon your unit's policy. If the wound is to be photographed it will be necessary to gain the patient's or their relative's written consent to do so.

To summarise, your documentation will include, measurements of the wound, classification of the wound's aetiology, the grade of the ulcer, appearance of the wound bed and skin surrounding it, exudate levels, any odour, any pain, type and frequency of dressing used and any further comments you feel appropriate. It is important that you gain the patient's consent to apply the dressings prior to any application.

CONCLUSION

As discussed, there are many grading systems that you may be expected to use during the course of your career. It is important that you are aware of how they all vary and familiarise yourself with your local grading system. You must document in your care plans which system you are using and if you are in any doubt about how it should be used then ask. The NICE guidelines (2003) clearly state that all healthcare professionals should receive training or education in pressure risk and assessment and that this should be interdisciplinary.

SELF-ASSESSMENT

After reading this chapter you should now take some time to reassess your knowledge base.

Reflection

Take some time to reflect upon the knowledge you have gained and how you will implement it into your own practice.

What knowledge did I possess prior to reading this chapter?

What do I know now?

How will my practice change as a result of attaining this knowledge?

Do I need to discuss with anyone practices I have witnessed that are not evidence-based, in relation to my new knowledge?

If so, who will I speak to?

Scenario

Complete this scenario based upon the knowledge you now possess.

Millie, a 17-year-old girl, has been admitted to your unit following a road traffic accident. She has an array of cuts and grazes over her body. She has a history of diabetes and her body mass index has indicated that she is overweight.

Tips on completing the scenario
Below is some information that you may have considered while working through the scenario. It is not an exhaustive list but it will give you some guidance on the information you should have collected.

You will need to make Millie as comfortable and as pain free as possible when she arrives on the ward. The road traffic accident has left her with an array of cuts and bruises that may all contain debris from the road. Therefore, these will require cleansing prior to you grading the wounds. The type of grading system needs to be chosen and this will largely depend on which one your unit or healthcare environments uses, that is, you will need to adhere to your local guidelines.

Chapter Three discussed the use of 'at risk' assessments; you will need to implement your local 'at risk' tool for Millie. Despite the fact that she is only 17 she may well be at risk of developing a pressure ulcer as she has been involved in a road traffic accident and she may be finding it difficult to move due to pain. Many of the 'at risk' tools provide you with a section that identifies any medical conditions which increase the risk of developing a pressure ulcer; these will include diabetes. You will need to ascertain if she suffers with Type I or Type II diabetes and document her normal diabetic regime. Her blood sugars will require careful and regular monitoring and must be documented in her care plan, with the medical staff being informed if there is a sudden drop or rise in them.

It may be useful to access and read the *National Service Framework for Diabetes* (DoH, 2003). Her weight will require recording and it will be necessary to record her body mass index and to perform a nutritional assessment on her.

Further areas for investigation
- A moving and handling assessment will require completion to ensure that safe techniques are used.
- Neurological assessment and observations.
- The importance of accurate documentation.
- Inclusion of the interdisciplinary team in her care. Personnel you may want to include will be: teachers; physiotherapists; occupational therapists; radiographers; paediatric nurses; tissue viability specialists; dieticians; pharmacists; medical staff and the pain team.

REFERENCES

David, J., Chapman, R. G., Chapman, E. G. & Lockett, B. (1983) *An Investigation of the Current Methods used in Nursing for the Care of Patients with Established Pressure Sores*. Nursing Practice Unit, Northwick Park, Middlesex.

Dealey, C. (1997) *Managing Pressure Sore Prevention*. Quay Books, Mark Allen Publishing Ltd, Salisbury.

Department of Health (2003) *National Service Framework for Diabetes*. Department of Health, London.

European Ulcer Advisory Panel (EPUAP) (1999) Guidelines on treatment of pressure ulcers. *Epuap Review*, **1**, 7–8.

Healey, F. (1995) The reliability and utility of pressure sore grading. *Journal of Tissue Viability*, **5** (40), 111–14.

Henderson, C. T., Ayello, E. A., Sussman, C., Leiby, D. M., Bennett, M. A., Dungog, E. F., Sprigle, S. & Woodruff, L. (1997) Draft definition of stage 1 pressure ulcers: inclusion of persons with darkly pigmented skin. NPUAP Task Force on Stage 1 Definition and Darkly Pigmented Skin. *Advances in Wound Care*, **10** (5), 16–19.

National Institute for Clinical Excellence (2003) *Pressure Ulcer Prevention. Pressure Ulcer Risk Assessment and Prevention; including the use of Pressure-relieving Devices (Beds, Mattresses and Overlays) for the Prevention of Pressure Ulcers in Primary and Secondary Care*. NICE Clinical guideline No 7. National Institute for Clinical Excellence, London. Available from: www.nice.org.uk

National Pressure Ulcer Advisory Panel (NPUAP) (1989) Pressure ulcer incidence, economics, risk assessment. Consensus development conference statement. *Decubitus*, **2** (2), 24–8.

Phillips, J. (1997) *Access to Clinical Education. Pressure Sores*. Churchill Livingstone, London.

Reid, J. & Morison, M. (1994) Towards consensus: classification of pressure sores. *Journal of Wound Care*, **3** (3), 157–60.

Torrance, C. (1983) *Pressure Sores, Aetiology, Treatment and Prevention*. Croom Helm, London.

6

Pressure Redistributing Devices and Equipment

INTRODUCTION

This chapter will discuss pressure redistributing devices that you may see being used within the clinical environments. Characteristics of a pressure redistributing device, how to choose a device for your patient and the various types of systems available for use will be identified and discussed.

LEARNING OBJECTIVES

By the end of this chapter the reader will be enabled to:

❏ Identify pressure redistributing devices
❏ Discuss the uses of various pressure redistributing devices
❏ Identify and discuss the criteria for choosing a pressure redistributing device
❏ Discuss how to care for the pressure redistributing device

Choice of equipment

There is an immense array and number of pressure redistributing devices on the market at present, over 200, with costs varying for their use, from a couple of pounds per day up to hundreds of pounds per day. With this amount of cost attributed to hiring, leasing or buying a piece of equipment it is important that the correct choice is made. Practical issues, such as the weight of the patient, may affect the choice of equipment. The company representatives will advise you as to which piece of equipment is suitable for the patient's weight. You should remember that you not only need to accurately ascertain the weight of the heavier patient, but also those patients who may be underweight, because the pressure exerted by the equipment may be too high and may lead to discomfort and possible skin damage. For those patients who are classed as obese, companies now produce a bariatric range of products suitable for weights over 225 kg. Furthermore, you will also need to assess the bed frame on which you are nursing your patient, as this too, will need to be able to accommodate the weight of the patient. Most bed frames will be suitable for a patient weighing up to 178 kg; anybody heavier will require a reinforced bed frame.

All healthcare professionals and people involved in administering nursing care to those patients who are at risk of developing a pressure ulcer, should be aware of the pressure redistributing systems available. They should be encouraged to promote the concept of prevention rather than treatment of pressure ulcers. It should be remembered that pressure area care does not only apply to those patients who are on prolonged bed rest, but also to those patients who may be required to sit in a chair for long periods of time; use a wheelchair; are on the operating table; or are on an accident and emergency trolley for a prolonged period of time. Those who suffer with reduced mobility are also at risk of skin damage. It is also worth noting that patients who sit out on a commode or on the toilet for long periods of time may be at risk of sustaining some pressure damage and, therefore, relief of pressure will be needed at regular intervals.

Who provides the equipment?

When you have assessed your patient and decided that a pressure redistributing device is required, it is necessary to find out who will be able to provide the chosen system.

Many trusts and healthcare centres will have a loan stores that you can contact and ask to provide you with the required equipment. You will be required to advise them of the patient's name and the location where the system is to be used, as the equipment will have been purchased or will be leased by your employer and they will need to keep track of the system. Some trusts and healthcare providers do not have a loan stores facility but do still purchase pressure redistributing equipment. If this is the case then the equipment may be in various areas throughout the healthcare area and you will need to contact the person responsible for allocating the equipment to ascertain where there is a piece of equipment currently not being used. Again, you will be asked to provide the patient details and location for the equipment you wish to loan. If your healthcare provider has not purchased any equipment they may well have a rental or leasing contract with a supplier. If the equipment is being leased there may be a loan stores. However, if the equipment is on a rental basis it will probably mean that you are required to telephone the suppliers directly, on an ad hoc basis, when you require a piece of equipment. If this is the case you must follow your local guidelines for renting a piece of equipment. Your loans store or supplier will be able to provide you with all types of pressure redistributing mattresses and cushions.

Wheelchair cushions

If you need a wheelchair cushion then there will be a specific person you will need to contact. This person may not be based in your own healthcare environment but may be in another acute trust or primary care trust. Wheelchair services exist in all health authorities, where patients can be assessed for suitable wheelchair cushions as well as wheelchairs. You will need to establish where your nearest provider is and a referral from a range of professionals, for example, physiotherapist, occupational therapist or qualified nurse will be required to acquire the cushion. When you have referred the patient for a cushion it is important that the wheelchair is available for the wheelchair specialist to see when providing the cushion, as all wheelchairs are different and patient needs are different. The cushion may be made to measure although many pressure care cushions come in a variety of sizes, which fit most standard wheelchairs. It must not affect the medical condition of the patient.

Remember that a decision as to whether or not a patient requires a piece of equipment must not be based solely upon the results of the assessment but also upon clinical judgement.

Characteristics of a pressure redistributing support system

When choosing a support system for a patient, certain characteristics should be taken into account. Ask yourself whether the support system:

- Distributes pressure evenly, provides frequent relief of pressure or constant low pressure?
- Conforms to body weight?
- Minimises friction and shearing forces?
- Provides a well ventilated, comfortable surface that does not unduly restrict movement?
- Maintains skin at a constant optimal temperature?
- Is acceptable to the patient?
- Does not impede care interventions and can quickly provide a hard surface for resuscitation procedures?
- Is easily cleaned and maintained?
- Is easily operated by both carers and patients?
- Has height adjustments, tilt facility, sufficient clearance for hoist use and is mobile with brakes?

(Torrance, 1983)

If the equipment does not fit these characteristics then it may be advisable to choose another product.

Why choose a specialised piece of equipment?

Assessment of the patient's condition and the type of pressure redistributing device required to meet their needs must be ongoing throughout their in-patient stay. If their condition improves or deteriorates then it may be necessary to review the equipment being utilised. What is accepted though, is that patients should not be placed on a standard foam mattress since they have been consistently outperformed by a range of foam-based low-pressure mattresses and overlays and by alternating pressure beds and mattresses. Although, the word 'standard' has varied in studies it is agreed that 'at risk' individuals should be placed on an alternative mattress to that of the hospital's standard foam mattress. Furthermore, patients who are undergoing surgery that have been identified as 'at risk' of developing a pressure ulcer should be nursed on a pressure redistributing mattress while undergoing surgery.

Results from randomised controlled tests have suggested that there is a reduction in post-operative pressure ulcers when an alternative support system has been used, rather than positioning the patient on a standard operating table. The NICE guidelines (2003) (Appendix Two) suggests that all individuals who are to undergo surgery and have been assessed as being vulnerable to pressure ulcer development should, as a minimum provision, be placed on either a high-specification foam theatre mattress or other pressure redistributing surfaces. It is interesting to note that there is no research evidence to suggest that high-tech pressure relieving mattresses and overlays are more effective than high specification (low-tech) foam mattresses and overlays. Professional consensus recommends that consideration should be given to the use of alternating pressure or other high-tech pressure relieving systems:

- As a first line prevention strategy for people at elevated risk as identified by holistic assessment
- When the individual's previous history of pressure ulcer prevention and/or clinical condition indicates that he/she is best cared for on a high-tech device
- When a low-tech device has failed (NICE, 2003. 1.2.4.3).

Seating

If a patient requires a pressure redistributing mattress then they will also require a pressure redistributing cushion for when they are sitting in a chair. The RCN (2001) suggested that any individuals who are considered to be acutely 'at risk' of developing pressure ulcers should restrict chair sitting to less than two hours until their general condition improves. This has been supported in the NICE guidelines (2003) (Appendix Two), which have stated that, even with appropriate pressure relief, it may be necessary to restrict sitting to less than two hours until the condition of the individual changes. Trained assessors, who possess the specific knowledge and expertise, should carry out seating assessments; these professionals are often the physiotherapist and/or the occupational therapist. When positioning an individual in a chair or wheelchair attention must be paid to the distribution of weight, postural alignment and foot support. There is a variety of seating pressure redistributing equipment available to choose from. However, none have been shown to outperform any other (NICE, 2003). Choice may well, then, be based upon individual preference or be dependent upon which company is supplying your trust with pressure redistributing equipment. Mattresses and cushions should be replaced as per the supplier's recommendations. Each mattress and cushion should be marked with the dates of purchase and regular checks should be made of their condition.

Maintaining integrity of the equipment

There are numerous tests to ascertain the condition of the equipment, that should be repeated regularly. This may be weekly if you can gain access to the equipment easily without compromising the safety of the patient. It is worth remembering that the Department of Health (2001, factors 6 and 7) (Appendix Three) recommend that the mattress be at least 130 mm in depth.

These tests include:

- Visual observation of the equipment – does the equipment look to be in good condition, are there any signs of deterioration, for example, staining of the covers, rips in the covers? If any faults are found they should be reported to the nurse in charge and removed from use. If there is a deterioration of the covers then this may be a focus for infection and they should be discarded and replaced.

- The hand compression test is where the tester will place both hands on the mattress and press down using their full body weight. It should be repeated for the entire length of the mattress and any variations in the density of the foam, including whether or not the base of the bed can be felt through the foam, should be recorded and reported. This phenomenon is commonly known as 'bottoming out'.

- The condition of the mattress should also be checked by unzipping the mattress cover and inspecting the condition of the foam. Please note that not all mattresses have a zip (to prevent leakage and deterioration to the foam). If this is the case you will need to check the company's recommendations.

- Some mattresses will require turning at regular intervals, for example, weekly, and this must be carried out to prolong the life of the equipment and to maintain the guarantee. Again, manufacturer's guidelines must be checked, as some equipment does not require turning.

- Equipment must be cleaned as per manufacturer's guidelines and when used with different patients, or when they become stained. Phenolics should NEVER be used as they cause mattress cover breakdown. As a rule soap and water is normally sufficient.

When assessing the mattress covers you must ensure that they possess the following qualities. They should be:

- Waterproof
- Water vapour permeable
- Fire retardant – they should meet the Medical Devices Agency standards and the British Standards Institute on fire retardancy

- Made from stretchable and durable material that is wrinkle free on the mattress

The mattress covers should have had these qualities when they were purchased. However, you may find that some mattress covers are rather old and did not meet these criteria when bought. These will require replacement with covers that meet the recommended standards or may require replacement of the whole mattress and cover.

Types of pressure redistributing support systems

The purpose of this section is to introduce the reader to the various types of pressure redistributing equipment. All the equipment identified will be referred to in generic terms and not by manufacturer's names. Pressure redistributing support systems can generally be placed into one of three groups, based upon their mode of operation.

Static
These systems seek to maximise the area of the patient's body in contact with the mattress surface, thereby reducing the magnitude of the contact pressure on any given anatomical location.

Dynamic
These systems include alternating pressure air mattresses that aim to vary systematically the anatomical locations of the body that bear weight, usually through the inflation and deflation of different sections of the support system. A pump controls the sequence of inflation and deflation. The systems are mains operated but many also have the capability of using battery power to allow for transfer between departments.

Turning
These systems systematically vary the body's centre of gravity and alter the loading upon specific anatomical points, through

the raising and lowering of the support system along its longitudinal axis. These systems tend to be used within a spinal unit environment (Morison, 2001).

Low-tech devices

These provide a conforming support surface that distributes the body weight over a large area (Cullum *et al.* 2001). They include the standard foam mattress, gel, fibre, fluid and air-filled mattresses and overlays. These are discussed in more detail later in this section.

High-tech devices

These are dynamic systems that include alternating pressure mattresses/overlays, air fluidised and low-air-loss beds, mattresses, overlays, and turning beds and frames (Cullum *et al.* 2001). These are discussed in more detail later in this section.

Pressure redistributing support surfaces are now widely used throughout the UK healthcare system, with a cost to the National Health Service of approximately £40 million annually, based upon the purchase and maintenance of the equipment. It is of great importance that the correct system is chosen for each patient and is reassessed at regular intervals. If you are unsure of how to choose the most appropriate system then advice should be sought from a practitioner who possesses knowledge of the various systems. It should be remembered that there are a lack of randomised controlled trials comparing the different support systems and inconsistent evidence relating to the effectiveness of static and dynamic support systems. Therefore, care must be taken when choosing a mattress. The equipment is NOT a substitute for good nursing care, repositioning or regular assessment of the patient's condition.

Overlays

A range of static mattress overlays are available, including fibre filled, foam, gel and air overlays. Fibre filled overlays often provide a great deal of comfort to the patient and do possess pressure redistributing capabilities. When the overlays are sent to the laundry, as they should be between use by each patient, the fibres become matted and damaged following the washing and drying procedures and the pressure redistributing capacity of the overlay is lost. Unfortunately, when they are returned to the ward they are still used.

Foam overlays are popular for low risk patients and provide pressure redistributing capabilities through the foam being cut to allow conformity to the patient's contours. However, there is a tendency for the foam to soften over time and no longer support the patient. Therefore, regular checking of these overlays for any signs of 'bottoming out' will be required. To increase the lifespan of this equipment you will need to turn the mattress weekly or as per manufacturer's guidelines.

Gel overlays are made of a thick deep gel that disperses pressure under the contours of the patient's body. The gel conducts the heat away from the user, thereby keeping it cooler for the user to sit or lie on. This type of overlay is mainly used within the operating theatre and accident and emergency departments of hospitals. These overlays are not as deep as the overlays you will see on the wards.

Air-filled overlays have been shown to produce the best interface pressure readings of all the overlays. These are normally alternating pressure overlays that allow the cells to inflate and deflate over a pre-prescribed timescale, thereby redistributing the pressure under the patient at regular intervals. These are also beneficial as the patient's bed can be transported between different departments without the mattress deflating. In addition, the alternation can be stopped to allow for cardiopulmonary resuscitation to be commenced if necessary. Also available is the low-air-loss overlay that constantly pumps air into the overlay. The mattress is made up of cells, which each have a small pin prick hole; when the patient's weight lies on the mattress the body weight allows the air to escape, allowing the surface to become softer and conform to the patient's body shape.

Replacement mattresses

These mattresses are used to replace the bed's original mattress. They may be comprised of foam of various densities; gel that also contains foam in addition to the cells of gel; alternating pressure air mattresses and low-air-loss mattresses. All claim to be effective for the prevention of pressure ulcers. It is your responsibility to accurately assess your patient and choose the most appropriate system for their needs. You will find that these mattresses all contain a two-way stretch cover.

Beds

Specialist bed systems are available for you to use. They tend to be expensive and therefore are often rented or leased rather than being bought from the manufacturer. The air-fluidised bed consists of a large tank filled with ceramic particles. Air flows constantly through the particles, providing a flotation effect. They are particularly useful for burns patients and those patients with heavily exuding wounds. Pressures are maintained at approximately 11 mmHg. As the air being circulated around the patient is continuously warm and dry their need for fluid replacement increases to an extra 1–1.5 litres per day.

Also available is the low-air-loss bed, which has a series of air sacs and constant airflow, maintaining pressures below 30 mmHg. The bed has electric controls, which the patient can use, if able and appropriate, for moving their position on the bed. In addition, some of the systems have scales incorporated into their design, allowing the patient to be weighed while on bed rest. Some of the more expensive designs have the ability to rotate or oscillate to improve respiratory function and, therefore, are particularly useful in an intensive therapy unit.

Turning beds or frames, also referred to as kinetic beds or kinetic therapy, are beds that aid manual repositioning of the patient by staff or aid in repositioning by motor driven turning or tilting.

Seating

It is important that you remember seating equipment when providing pressure redistributing equipment for your patients. Patients can, and will, develop pressure ulcers when sitting in a chair for a prolonged period of time. When you look around clinical areas you will note a variety of designs and sizes of chairs. A patient should be assessed for the correct height and type of chair. For example, a patient who has undergone a total hip replacement will require a high chair to prevent dislocation of the hip prosthesis and not a low chair. This, as well as pressure redistributing qualities, will need to be taken into account when choosing the chair. The chair should also be in good condition, with no tears in the covering that may be a focus for infection. When the patient is seated their feet should reach the ground and they should not be 'slumped' in the chair. If the patient is constantly slipping down the chair this will lead to a risk of shear and friction injuries. Positioning of individuals who spend substantial periods of time in a chair or wheelchair should take into account: distribution of weight, postural alignment and support of feet (NICE, 2003, 1.2.2.3). You may find it helpful to employ the skills of the physiotherapist or occupational therapist to assess your patient for the correct chair. Indeed, the RCN (2001), state that: 'seating assessments for aids and equipment should be carried out by trained assessors who have the specific knowledge and expertise'. Many of the pressure redistributing systems companies will undertake a chair and seating audit for you on request, where they will identify any equipment that requires replacement.

Pressure redistributing cushions are available for seating and wheelchairs, and should be used as appropriate. A specialist should assess wheelchair users for a cushion; this may be a physiotherapist or occupational therapist. It should be mentioned that there is very little research or random controlled trials that support or dispute the use of the various types of pressure redistributing cushions. However, you should consider that over 50% of body weight is supported on 8% of the sitting area (that is to say, at or near the ischial tuberosoities) and the use of a cushion will have a direct effect on the effectiveness of the chair you have chosen for your patient, as it will alter the position of the armrests and the seat height. Please ensure that you do seek advice prior to their use. Each cushion, as with the mattresses, should have a vapour permeable two-way stretch cover and under no circumstances should you place another covering over the cushions, for example, a pillowcase, as these are a cause of friction and undermine the properties of the cushions. Before using a cushion for your patient check that it will not have an adverse effect on the patient's medical condition, for example, patients who have undergone spinal surgery or major joint replacement may have specific medical instructions on what position and at what height they may sit.

The cushions you may see in a care setting may be:

- *Fibre filled*, which unfortunately would appear to deteriorate over a short period of time and tend to be used for patient comfort rather than their pressure redistributing abilities.
- *Foam filled* that are available in a variety of thickness with various levels of foam density. The different densities tend to allow for heavier weights to be supported. Costs of the cushions will also vary depending upon the density of the foam.
- *Alternating cushions*: these cushions alternate under the patient through rows of cells that inflate and deflate over a regular period to aid in the redistribution of pressure.

Interestingly, the NICE (2003) guidelines state that no seat cushion has been shown to perform better than another. This has led to them being unable to recommend a specific type of cushion for pressure redistribution purposes (Appendix Two). The choice of cushion for your patient will, therefore, be dependent upon local guidelines. The *Essence of Care* document (DoH, 2001), sections on pressure ulcers, factors 6 and 7, will provide you with some guidance on choosing the most appropriate piece of equipment (Appendix Three). In addition, the NICE guidelines (2003) provides guidance on the most effective use of devices.

What not to use!
The following should NOT be used as pressure reducing aids:

- Water filled gloves are ineffective under heels because the small surface area of the heel means it is not possible to redistribute the pressure by this localised method.
- Synthetic sheepskins provide no pressure reducing properties. Some individuals may wish to use them for comfort, in which case care must be taken when laundering and with regard too cross infection. Document in your nursing notes that the patient has requested to use this equipment.
- Doughnut type devices are believed to adversely affect lymphatic drainage and circulation and cause rather than prevent pressure ulcer formation.
- Mattresses that are below 130 mm in depth (except for trolley mattresses).

The NICE (2003) guidelines provide further information on this subject (Appendix Two).

Education
Bennett (1995) stated that the cost of wound management is £1 billion per annum in the UK, and this figure does not take into account litigation costs, which are becoming more common in nursing practice (Tingle, 1991.) This fact, in conjunction with recommendations made by the UKCC to expand professional roles to promote improved patient care (UKCC, 2000), has focused the attention of many nurses upon the importance of continuing educational development to ensure that their practice is supported by up-to-date research and evidence. It is important that all staff involved in the prevention of pressure ulcers are up-to-date with techniques and

understand the possible causes and treatments of pressure ulcer development. There are many guidelines available for staff to refer to that include those produced by the National Institute for Clinical Excellence (2003) and the *Essence of Care* (DoH, 2001) (Appendices Two and Three). Patients and their relatives/carers should also be educated in the importance of protecting their pressure areas and understanding how to prevent breakdown.

The NICE guidelines (2003) are quite explicit in how they recommend education and training for pressure ulcer prevention. They state that healthcare professionals with recognised training in pressure ulcer management should cascade their knowledge and skills to their local healthcare teams. Furthermore, an interdisciplinary approach to the training and education of healthcare professionals should be adopted. Box 6.1 highlights the content of a training and education programme as recommended in the NICE (2003) guidelines.

It should be remembered that *The Patients Charter* (DoH, 1995) recommended that while patients are in hospital they should be cared for in a safe environment with reasonable established measures to ensure their safety. Additionally, the *Code of Professional Conduct* (NMC, 2002) stated that nurses are personally accountable for their practice. You are therefore answerable for any actions and omissions, regardless of advice or directions from another professional. You have a duty of care to your patients and clients, who are entitled to receive safe and competent care. Furthermore, the NMC (2002) stated that nurses must keep their knowledge and skills up-to-date throughout their working life. In particular, inclusion in learning activities that develop competence and performance should be undertaken at regular intervals, which obviously relates directly to education relevant to tissue viability activities and knowledge.

Box 6.1 Recommended training and education programme content.

- Risk factors for pressure ulcer development
- Pathophysiology of pressure ulcer development
- Limitations and potential applications of risk assessment tools
- Skin assessments
- Skin care
- Selection of pressure redistributing equipment
- Use of pressure redistributing equipment
- Maintenance of pressure redistributing equipment
- Methods of documenting risk assessments and prevention activities
- Positioning to minimise pressure
- Shear and friction damage, including the correct use of manual handling devices
- Roles and responsibilities of interdisciplinary team members in pressure ulcer management
- Policies and procedures regarding transferring individuals between care settings, and patient education and information gathering
- Providing education and information to patients

Reproduced with kind permission from the National Institute for Clinical Excellence (2003) *Pressure Ulcer Prevention. Pressure Ulcer Risk Assessment and Prevention; including the use of Pressure-relieving Devices (Beds, Mattresses and Overlays) for the Prevention of Pressure Ulcers in Primary and Secondary Care.* NICE Clinical Guideline No 7. National Institute for Clinical Excellence, London. Available from: www.nice.org.uk

Patients and carers also need education and training in the prevention of pressure ulcer prevention. Many patients on discharge home may be alone or be reliant on carers to help them change position and to maintain their activities of daily living. The NICE (2003) guidelines offer advice on what education should be provided to patients and carers. These can be viewed in Box 6.2 below.

Box 6.2 Recommended patient/carer education.

- The risk factors associated with developing a pressure ulcer
- The sites that are of greatest risk of pressure damage
- How to inspect skin and recognise skin changes
- How to care for skin
- Methods for pressure relief/reduction
- Where to seek further advice and assistance should they need it
- The need for immediate visits to a healthcare professional should signs of damage be noticed

Reproduced with kind permission from the National Institute for Clinical Excellence (2003) *Pressure Ulcer Prevention. Pressure Ulcer Risk Assessment and Prevention; including the use of Pressure-relieving Devices (Beds, Mattresses and Overlays) for the Prevention of Pressure Ulcers in Primary and Secondary Care.* NICE Clinical Guideline No 7. National Institute for Clinical Excellence, London. Available from: www.nice.org.uk

---

CONCLUSION

This chapter has discussed the use of a variety of pressure redistributing equipment, how to choose a piece of equipment and how to maintain its integrity. It is not an exhaustive list and, where appropriate, advice may be sought from the tissue viability specialist, equipment coordinator or the company representatives supplying the equipment. It is important that you remember that the equipment is not a replacement for good individualised nursing care. Any equipment you use must be documented and a risk assessment must have been carried out prior to its implementation.

SELF-ASSESSMENT

After reading this chapter you should now take some time to reassess your knowledge base. You should now be able to identify various pressure redistributing devices and discuss the differences between them. In addition, you should be able to discuss the importance of using appropriate devices following reassessment of the patient's needs.

Reflection

Take some time to reflect upon the knowledge you have gained and how you will implement it into your own practice.

What knowledge did I possess prior to reading this chapter?

What do I know now?

How will my practice change as a result of attaining this knowledge?

Do I need to discuss with anyone practices I have witnessed that are not evidence-based, in relation to my new knowledge?

If so, who will I speak to?

Scenario

Joyce is an 82-year-old lady who lived alone prior to being admitted to your ward. She had been found on her front room floor by a neighbour 14 hours after having tripped over a rug. On admission you document that she is a large lady, weighing 165 kg, whose mobility has been declining for the past six months, leaving her housebound. You also note that she has a 2 cm by 4 cm superficial break to her sacrum and a red, soft area to her left heel.

Tips on completing the scenario
Below is some information that you may have considered while working through the scenario. It is not an exhaustive list but it will give you some guidance on the information you should have collected.

As Joyce is overweight, has compromised skin integrity and an established wound on admission, you will need to consider which pressure redistributing devices will meet her needs. You will need to ensure that the pieces of equipment chosen will withhold her weight. As she is under 178 kg, she will not require a reinforced bed frame. Joyce will require a pressure redistributing cushion in addition to a mattress, for the periods of time when she sits out of bed. You must ensure that the chair is the correct height for her when the cushion is placed on it. You may want to refer to the NICE guidelines for this advice.

When choosing your piece of equipment you need to ensure that Joyce consents to be nursed on it and that it is comfortable for her. You will need to ensure that it meets the characteristics of an ideal pressure redistributing device as described in the chapter.

You will need to undertake an assessment of her activities of daily living and perform a variety of assessments on Joyce that will include:

- Moving and handling
- Nutritional
- Pain
- 'At risk'

All the results will need to be documented in her care plan with reassessment dates.

Further areas for investigation
Appropriate wound dressings will need to be examined (see Chapter Seven).

REFERENCES

Bennett, G. (1995) *Wound Care for Health Professionals*. 2nd edn. Chapman and Hall, London.

Cullum, N., Nelson, E. A., Flemming, K. and Sheldon, T. (2001) Systematic reviews of wound care management: (5) beds; (6) compression; (7) laser therapy, therapeutic ultrasound, electrotherapy and electromagnetic therapy. *Health Technology Assessment*, **5** (9). www.ncchta.org/pdfexecs/summ509.pdf. Accessed 15 May 2004.

Department of Health (1995) *The Patients Charter and You*. HMSO, London.

Department of Health (2001) *Essence of Care. Patient Focused Benchmarking for Healthcare Practitioners*. Department of Health, London.

Morison, M. (2001) *The Prevention and Treatment of Pressure Ulcers*. Mosby, London.

National Institute for Clinical Excellence (2003) *Pressure Ulcer Prevention. Pressure Ulcer Risk Assessment and Prevention; including the Use of Pressure-relieving Devices (Beds, Mattresses and Overlays) for the Prevention of Pressure Ulcers in Primary and Secondary Care*. NICE Clinical guideline No 7. National Institute for Clinical Excellence, London. Available from www.nice.org.uk

Nursing and Midwifery Council (2002) *Code of Professional Conduct*. Nursing and Midwifery Council, London.

Royal College of Nursing (2001) *Pressure Ulcer Risk Assessment and Prevention Recommendations*. NICE Guidelines. Royal College Nursing, London.

Tingle, J. H. (1991) Accountability and the law: how it affects the nurse. *Senior Nurse*, **10** (2), 8–9.

Torrance, C. (1983) *Pressure Sores: Aetiology, Treatment and Prevention*. Croom Helm, London.

United Kingdom Central Council for Nursing, Midwifery and Health Visiting (2000) *Fitness for Practice*. United Kingdom Central Council for Nursing, London.

7

Management of the Established Pressure Ulcer

This chapter will discuss the principles and nursing care associated with the management of an established pressure ulcer. In addition, it will discuss methods of debridement, cleansing of a wound, types of dressings and how to choose the most appropriate dressings. Finally, you will be asked to reflect on what you have learnt and a case study will be presented that you are encouraged to undertake.

It will be useful for you to revisit the information and guidance contained in Appendix Three at this stage. This will allow you to identify the following benchmarks:

- Appropriate screening and assessment (Factor 1)
- Who undertakes the assessment (Factor 2)
- Informing patients/clients and carers (Factor 3)
- Individualised plan for the prevention and treatment of pressure ulcers (Factor 4)

LEARNING OBJECTIVES
By the end of this chapter the reader will be enabled to:

❏ Discuss which issues require consideration when planning the care of a patient with an established pressure ulcer
❏ Identify the microbiological state of a wound
❏ Identify different types of wounds
❏ Identify various wound dressings
❏ Discuss how to cleanse and dress a wound effectively

INTRODUCTION

There are times when a patient will develop a pressure ulcer while in your care, or who is admitted to your care with an established pressure ulcer, despite preventative measures being undertaken. If the patient is admitted with a pressure ulcer, then it is vital that you document this in your nursing notes, stating the size, grade and position of the ulcer and treatment being used on admission. If you change the treatment plan the rationale for this will also require documentation. It will be your responsibility to make available a plan of care to treat the ulcer and administer holistic care to that patient. Your plan of care will need to include assessing the patient's needs and choosing not only the most appropriate dressing, but also the appropriate pressure redistributing device and ensuring that the patient is nutritionally stable. Choosing the appropriate pressure redistributing device has been discussed in Chapter Six and I advise you to revisit this chapter. Your goal when treating and managing the established pressure ulcer is to maintain a warm, moist wound-healing environment facilitating the healing process. It is pertinent to point out that it will not always be possible for you to heal that wound completely. It may be necessary to refer the patient to a surgeon for reconstructive surgery to help promote integrity of the skin.

During the assessment process of the patient's pressure ulcer you will need to grade the ulcer accurately. It is important that you use your workplace's recognised grading system and that it is documented in the patient's care plan, ensuring that all staff use the same tool. It is worth mentioning that if the patient is admitted to your unit from another hospital or care environment they may well have had their ulcer graded using a different tool from your own; therefore, the numbers assigned to each category may vary. You should make a note of this during the first assessment and document the tool you will be using while the patient is in your care. It may be helpful for you to refer to Appendix Three, the *Essence of Care* guidelines for pressure ulcers (DoH, 2001) Factor 4, that provides the benchmark for individualised plans of prevention and treatment of pressure ulcers. As discussed in Chapter One, it is now accepted that a moist, warm environment is the most effective situation in which to heal a wound. Therefore, the cleansing agents and wound dressings you choose for your patient should maintain this type of environment.

Planning the care

When planning the care of a patient with an established pressure ulcer, you must remember that your plan of care is not just about choosing the correct dressing but should encompass the holistic needs of the patient. It should also take into account many additional factors, some of which will now be discussed.

Nutritional state

As mentioned in previous chapters adequate nutrition is vital to the prevention and management of pressure ulcers. If a patient is nutritionally impaired than this will prevent the ulcer from healing. The diet needs to contain proteins, fats, carbohydrates, vitamins and minerals; therefore, referral to the dietician will be appropriate if dietary intake is a concern.

Information and guidance regarding the importance of food and nutrition is presented in the *Essence of Care* document (DoH, 2001). There are ten factors that are presented and the author recommends that you access this section of the document to enable you to understand the benchmarks relevant to the importance of adequate nutrition. The full document can be accessed via the Internet at the following address: www.doh.gov.uk/essenceofcare

Carbohydrates

As the body attempts to heal the ulcer, there will be an increase in the requirements for carbohydrates, due to the increase in the metabolic rate. The carbohydrates will be broken down and will provide glucose, which is an important source of energy.

Proteins

The demand for proteins will also increase, with collagen being the main protein synthesised: in periods of stress or sepsis the need for proteins will increase. These proteins are required in the inflammatory stage and to allow the wound-healing process to progress to the granulation stage. A lack of proteins may cause the wound to remain in the inflammatory stage for an extended period of time. If protein depletion is severe then development of oedema may be witnessed, due to hypoalbuminaemia affecting the rate and quality of healing.

Vitamins

Patients will require a variety of vitamins to help maintain a successful wound-healing regime. These include vitamin C that helps to synthesis collagen and to form bands of collagen fibres and provide wound strength. Vitamin K helps to form thrombin to prevent the formation of a haematoma. Vitamins A and B aid in the cross-linking of collagen.

Minerals

Minerals have an important role to play in the wound-healing process. Zinc is required for protein synthesis and helps to prevent bacterial growth. Iron helps to maintain the oxygen supply to the wound site and copper is a cofactor in the synthesis of collagen.

Documenting nutritional intake

It is clear that nutrition is important and you must keep accurate records of the patient's nutritional assessments and dietary intake. It may also be necessary for the patient to have blood taken for biochemistry tests. Medical staff may prescribe supplements to enhance the patient's diet, yet there is little evidence to support that this achieves any better clinical outcomes.

The most important aspect of your role as a nurse is to ensure that the patient receives a well balanced diet that they enjoy and you record their nutritional intake daily. It may be useful to complete a food record chart during their in-patient stay. This will normally occur over a 24-hour period and will allow you to assess the amount of proteins, fats, energy, minerals, vitamins and fluids consumed by the patient over that period of time. It is only a snapshot of their dietary intake but will give you some baseline information on which you can plan their care. Indeed, the Department of Health (2001) states that, the amount of food the patient actually eats should be monitored and recorded and action taken if there is a cause for concern.

Assessing the patient's weight

Daily weight recordings of the patient provide a guideline to excessive weight loss. Thomas (1994) stated that a weight loss of 10% or more during the preceding three months should be considered as a cause for concern. A record of the patient's body mass index (BMI) will provide you with an indication of their nutritional status. The BMI is a method of calculating body weight that takes into account the patient's body weight and their height. It is not one hundred per cent accurate but will allow some form of baseline measurement to assess whether the patient is underweight or overweight. The dieticians may also use skin fold measurements or total body fat measurements to formulate a more accurate assessment.

The BMI can be calculated as:

$$BMI = \frac{Weight\,(kg)}{Height\,(m)^2}$$

Table 7.1 Classification of BMI.

Under 20 – underweight
20–24 – healthy weight
25–29 – overweight
Over 30 – obese
Over 40 – very obese

The BMI classification is demonstrated in Table 7.1. It is important to be aware that the BMI is not one hundred per cent accurate and that a patient who presents with a high BMI may in fact be malnourished, but the presence of oedema has distorted the weight recording.

Remember, it is of no use to provide the patient with a nutritionally strong meal if they do not like the food you have presented to them. It is necessary to ensure that during their nutritional assessment you have made a note of their likes and dislikes and that the diet ordered for them reflects this information. The Department of Health (2001, Factors 1, 2, 4, 5, 6, 7, 9 and 10) suggest that patients, relatives and carers should be given sufficient information to enable them to obtain their food and that the plan of care is based upon ongoing nutritional assessments that are devised, implemented and evaluated regularly.

Dehydration

Dehydration will lead to an electrolyte imbalance and in turn will impair cellular function. It is important that you ensure that your patient is drinking adequate amounts and if not, it may be necessary to commence intravenous fluids. An accurate fluid balance chart should be maintained. Patients and their families/carers should be made aware that a fluid balance chart is in progress, and that to ensure its accuracy they too should chart any drinks that are consumed by the patient.

Stress

People who are admitted to a healthcare environment are often anxious and worried, particularly if they have a pressure ulcer or any other type of wound. Anxiety causes the release of glucocorticoids that have an anti-inflammatory effect and inhibit fibroblasts, collagen synthesis and formation of granulation tissue. To help prevent this, effective communication with the patient and their families, explaining all procedures, will be useful and if necessary they can be offered the services of a counsellor.

Medication

Some types of medication will have an adverse effect on wound healing, including steroid treatment, anti-inflammatory medication, cytotoxic drugs, immunosuppressive drugs and anticoagulants, by interrupting either cell division or the clotting process. You must document all the patient's medications and use this information in your assessments.

Radiotherapy and chemotherapy

These will inhibit cell division and suppress cell growth.

Lack of rest

Rest and sleep are necessary for wound healing as tissue repair and the rate of cellular division are enhanced by sleep. You must try and promote rest and sleep for patients with wounds.

Ageing process

As age advances we have a reduction in the activity of fibroblasts, causing wound contraction and epithelialisation to slow down, with the immune system becoming less effective, therefore taking the skin longer to repair. The older the person is the more likely they are to have associated diseases that may impinge upon the healing process. These may include conditions such as cardiac disease and chronic breathing problems, that all reduce the supply of oxygen to the wound. Diseases such as rheumatoid arthritis may cause ulceration. Morison and Moffatt (1997) identified that 10% of leg ulcers were detected in people suffering with rheumatoid arthritis. Also remember that people who suffer with a loss of sensation or movement, for example, from spinal injuries, fractures or cerebrovascular accident will be at increased risk of pressure ulcer development, as they will be unaware of pain or a loss of sensation occurring.

Diabetes mellitus

People diagnosed with diabetes mellitus will require extra care of their wounds and extra observation of the 'at risk' areas. Diabetes is linked to peripheral neuropathy and arteriosclerosis, which can both lead to ulceration. Patients and families/carers should also be educated regarding the risks of damage to skin integrity caused by diabetes. Referral to the diabetic nurse specialist will be helpful and they will be able to offer advice to nursing staff and the patients and relatives.

Wound management

A failure to correctly assess and treat wounds will lead to a failure to heal. It is important that a competent practitioner undertakes the assessment process and plans the care. If in doubt, ASK! If you are a qualified practitioner, you are accountable for your own actions and omissions; it is up to you as a professional to seek out the knowledge you require prior to undertaking any procedure. The Nursing and Midwifery Council (NMC) (2002, 1.3) quite clearly states: 'You are personally accountable for your practice. This means that you are answerable for your actions and omissions, regardless of advice or directions from another professional.'

If you are new to treating pressure ulcers or other areas of tissue viability, you must ensure that you are competent to undertake the procedure and that you have received the correct training. You must not feel pressurised to undertake any procedure that you do not feel capable to undertake even if your ward or unit is very busy at the time. The NMC (2002, 1.4) reminds you that: 'You have a duty of care to your patients and clients, who are entitled to receive safe and competent care.'

If you are unsure then ask to be educated on the issue and observe another practitioner undertaking the procedure. Ask them their rationale for planning the care.

Psychological problems

The presence of a wound may cause psychological distress to some patients. Therefore, effective communication between you and your patient is vital. If necessary, counselling services may be required, with discussions relating to altered body image. The family and carers should be involved in these discussions, with the patient's permission. Smoking, alcohol and drug dependency all affect the healing rate and patients should be discouraged from these activities. In addition, smoking impairs healing by reducing oxygen availability to damaged tissues. Education regarding the risks of smoking should be offered to the patient and referral to smoking cessation sessions may be appropriate if the patient agrees.

Social factors

The Black Report (1982) identified that people in the lowest of the five social groupings were almost twice as likely to become ill than those in the highest group. This suggests that there is a strong link between social circumstance and health. Indeed, it has been noted that people from a lower social grouping tend to eat less nutritious meals. If, during the assessment process, social factors are identified as an issue that may prevent wound healing, it may be necessary to offer health promotion advise to the patient and their family. It may also be appropriate to send a referral to the social worker who may be able to advise on extra benefits for the family.

Wound history

It is important that you ascertain how the wound or ulcer occurred. For example, has the patient had a pressure ulcer previously, was it in the same area, what was the treatment and how effective was the treatment plan in healing the ulcer? Your findings will need to be documented and the plan of care should reflect any past treatments. It may also be useful to contact the practitioners who were treating the ulcer previously, to discuss the care. When you have completed the assessment and produced a plan of care you may then cleanse the wound. This procedure will now be discussed.

Cleansing the wound

The main objective for cleansing a wound is to remove any foreign matter or debris that may impair the wound-healing process. Wounds should only be cleansed when they are dirty, with either warm normal saline or tap water, and not on a daily basis. As a rule you will need to cleanse the wound if there are any visible signs of debris after the initial wound has occurred or if the ulcer is contaminated with bodily fluids, for example, if the ulcer is a sacral pressure ulcer. You may need to cleanse the wound/ulcer to remove excess slough and exudate or to remove any remaining dressing material. Always ask yourself: why am I cleansing this wound? If you cannot offer a rational explanation to the question do not cleanse. It is important that you do warm your cleansing solution prior to application to the wound, as tissue hypothermia, caused by introducing a cool or cold solution to the wound bed, can result in decreased mitogenesis and decreased phagocyte activity. It can take as long as 40 minutes for a wound to regain its original temperature after cleansing and several hours for cellular activity to return to normal (Flanagan, 1997). Minimal mechanical force should be used and cotton wool balls should never be used, as they will leave particles behind, causing a focus for infection. Cavity wounds should be cleansed using irrigation.

When applying the cleansing solution you should not use excessive force, but just enough to remove the debris and not enough to damage the viable tissue. Ovington (2001) states that a safe range of effective irrigation pressures has been established as 27.6–103.5 kPa (4–15 psi). A 35 ml syringe fitted with a 19-gauge angiocatheter tip will deliver a stream of liquid at a pressure of 55.2 kPa (8 psi). Increasing the bore of the angiocatheter or decreasing the size of the syringe results in higher pressure streams, whereas decreasing the bore or increasing the size of the syringe results in lower pressures. Remember, patients may be encouraged to take showers, which will not only cleanse the wound but will also make the patient feel clean.

You may hear three terms referred to regarding the microbiological state of the wounds you are caring for in the clinical areas. These are: contamination, colonisation and infection. It is important that you understand the meaning of these terms and the differences between the three.

Contamination   This is characterised by the presence of micro-organisms in the wound, without proliferation, and it is generally accepted that all wounds are contaminated. This means that no wounds are sterile (Williams and Leaper, 1998).

Colonisation   This is a common condition in chronic wounds and does not necessarily affect the healing process. In colonisation there is a presence and proliferation of micro-organisms.

Infection   In this state the bacteria invade the healthy tissue and continue to proliferate, eventually taking over the host immune response. You will be able to observe this reaction easily by looking at the wound and noting local redness, swelling, odour, bleeding, bridging, pocketing, cessation of healing, and changes in the amount and colour of the exudate. In addition, the patient may well complain of pain and present with a pyrexia.

The use of antiseptics and antibiotics

The EPUAP (1999) recommend that antiseptics should not be routinely used. However, they may be considered when clinical assessment suggests that bacterial loads need to be controlled and in this case should only be used for a limited time, until the wound is clean and the inflammation reduced. The emergence of infections such as Methicillin Resistant Staphylococcus Aureus (MRSA) has led many hospitals and healthcare centres to develop in-depth policies, protocols and guidelines regarding the treatment of these infections and which antiseptics may and may not be used in the treatment of chronic wounds. Many writers have argued that, in the past, widespread use of topical antibiotics in wound care has contributed to the evolution of these infections. However, there have also been positive results reported for the use of topical antibiotics in acute wounds. You are strongly advised to seek these out and if necessary discuss them with your infection control team. If you use an antiseptic on a wound, remember that these antiseptics not only work by destroying the bacterial cell walls, but also by destroying the non-bacterial cells such as the fibroblasts. Also remember that effective and correct hand washing techniques by all members of the interdisciplinary team will help to prevent the spread of infection.

Debridement

Some wounds which you observe may require debridement prior to treating the wound, that is to say, the wound requires the removal of devitalised (dead) tissue. It is important that the person who debrides the wound has been taught how to undertake the procedure and feels competent to do it. Devitalised tissue will delay wound healing and will predispose the wound to colonisation and may lead to infection. Therefore, it is important that it is removed to provide an optimal healing environment. You will be able to recognise a wound that requires debridement by its appearance. It may be necrotic or have yellow slough, and there are various techniques to remove it. These include *sharp debridement*, using scissors or a scalpel, and can be performed in an outpatient's clinic or on the wards. In severe cases a surgeon in an operating theatre may perform it. *Mechanical debridement* involves using wet to dry dressings, high-pressure irrigation or scrubbing of the wound, but this may damage the wound bed. *Enzymatic removal* involves using moisture retentive dressings and *autolytic debridement* involves using moisture retentive dressings that retain the endogenous enzymes at the wound surface, thus digesting the devitalised tissue. Whichever techniques are used, a competent appropriately trained practitioner must undertake the procedure. If in doubt do NOT undertake the procedure, and as rule student nurses should NOT be attempting this procedure.

The EPUAP (1999) has offered quite clear guidelines on wound debridement as shown in Box 7.1.

Box 7.1 European Pressure Ulcer Advisory Panel guidelines on wound debridement (EPUAP, 1999).

- Remove devitalised tissue when appropriate for the patient's condition and consistent with the patient's goals.
- Methods of debridement include surgical, enzymatic, autolytic, larvae or a combination.
- Surgical, enzymatic or autolytic debridement techniques may be used when there is no urgent clinical need for drainage or removal of devitalised tissue. If there is an urgent need for debridement it must be performed by a competent person.
- Overall quality of life and the manner in which to accomplish debridement must be taken into account when treating a wound in the terminally ill person.
- Surgical methods include scissors, scalpel, that may be used by a nurse at the bedside, or surgical debridement performed by a surgeon in the operating theatre.
- Pain associated with surgical debridement should be prevented or managed.

- Dry eschar need not be debrided if oedema, erythema or drainage are not present.
- Dry eschar may be removed using dressings, for example, hydrocolloids and/or hydrogels.
- Wounds should be assessed daily for any changes and the results documented.

Reproduced with kind permission from the European Pressure Ulcer Advisory Panel.

Types of wound

You need to be aware of the types of wound that you may be expected to treat prior to choosing a dressing. These may be classified as:

- **Necrotic** (black) – the aims are to debride and remove the eschar, provide the right environment for autolysis and to assess the wound depth and exudate levels.
- **Sloughy** (yellow) – the aims are to liquefy and remove the slough, preparing the wound bed for granulation and to be able to assess the wound depth and exudate levels.
- **Infected** (green) – the aims are to reduce the exudates and odour, and to promote healing, while treating the wound symptomatically and changing the dressings daily.
- **Granulating** (red) – the aim is to support the granulation process by protecting new tissue and maintaining a warm, moist environment.
- **Epithelialising** (pink) – the aim is to provide suitable conditions for resurfacing of the wound and to disturb the wound as infrequently as possible.

The next section of this chapter is dedicated to identifying the dressings available on the market. The following list is not exhaustive and the author suggests you contact your tissue viability specialist to discuss dressings used in your area. However, it will give you an insight into the number of different dressing types available to choose from. Your own area of work may have a contract for the provision of dressings and it is important to ascertain which dressings you are recommended to use. If you require one that is not provided by the contract or recommended on your formulary then you will need to establish the procedure to acquire it.

Dressings

There are a variety of wound dressings available on the market for practitioners to choose from, which can often be a confusing process. It is vital that you understand what each dressing does and understand the rationale and research underpinning the use of these dressings. A wound dressing is a form of medication and you must be aware of its properties prior to application to a wound.

Flanagan and Fletcher (2003, p. 183) identify two main categories of dressing products: passive and interactive. They describe passive dressings as products that have no direct effect on the wound. These dressings have little absorbency and become saturated quickly, often leading to leakage and the dressing falling off the wound. In wounds that have a small amount of exudate, the dressing becomes dry and thus it becomes painful and traumatic to remove it. However, these products are of use in wounds with minimal or no drainage, or as a secondary dressing. They describe interactive dressings as providing the optimum environment at the wound interface. These products may be occlusive or semi-occlusive. However, not all of them contain these properties. In addition, they highlight that many manufacturers are now developing dressings that combine the two groups, thus offering the benefits of both categories.

The following section will describe a selection of the wound dressing products you may witness but remember that this is not an exhaustive list of the available products.

Alginates

These dressings are extracted from various varieties of seaweeds. They are highly absorbent and suitable for moderate to heavily exuding wounds. They should be applied to the wound dry, as on contact with the wound exudate they form a gel, absorbing the exudate, debriding the slough and encouraging granulation of the wound. They can be used on infected wounds and it is recommended that they are changed every 2–3 days or twice a week as healing progresses. These dressings require moisture to function and are not suitable for dry wounds or wounds covered with black eschar. Alginates are available in two forms: a flat sheet and rope type, which is suitable for cavity wounds.

Bio-surgery

This is larvae therapy, or the use of maggots. They should be used on infected or necrotic wounds, and as a rule should not be used in the treatment of a fistula or wounds that may connect with vital organs. Patient consent must be sought and it may be necessary to offer counselling to the patient and/or relatives/carers prior to, and during, their application. The maggots should be applied as per the manufacturer's guidelines. A competent relevant trained practitioner, normally the tissue viability specialist or a wound care link nurse, should undertake the procedure of application of the larvae.

Carbon wound dressings

Carbon dressings are beneficial for controlling odour and some contain silver that destroys the bacteria.

Foam dressings

These may be used as a primary or secondary dressing, helping to maintain a moist, warm, healing environment. They are suitable for low to moderately exuding wounds, but are not useful on dry or superficial wounds, or those covered with a scab or hard necrotic tissue. They may be used for flat or cavity wounds. Exudate from the wound is absorbed into the dressing and drawn away from the wound, helping to prevent maceration. Foam dressings are available as adhesive or non-adhesive with the adhesive being deactivated on contact with moisture, therefore causing no pain to the patient on removal. These dressings may be cut to conform to the wound shape.

Hydrocolloids

These dressings remain extremely popular within the clinical areas, with a variety of manufacturers producing different forms of the dressings. The dressings interact with wound exudate by absorbing fluid to form a gel and are waterproof. They are suitable for desloughing and for light to medium exuding wounds and may be left in place for up to seven days. They should not be used in patients with an anaerobic infection. When applying the dressings it is worth noting that they should be warmed in your hand for 3–5 minutes prior to application to make the dressing pliable and then sealed in place by using the warmth of your hands. Remember to leave a 1.5–2 cm margin around the edges of the wound when applying the dressing. This will allow for the gelling action of the dressing. This type of product tends to give off a characteristic odour when being changed, caused by the gelatin and pectin content. These products may not be acceptable to vegans so check with the patient prior to application (Stringfellow *et al.* 2003).

Hydrofibre dressings

These are highly absorbent dressings made from non-woven pads or ribbon dressings containing hydrocolloid fibres. They convert from a dry dressing to a soft gel on contact with moisture, drawing up and retaining exudate fluid and debris within the fibres. The dressings promote angiogenesis and aid autolytic debridement of the wound. They are effective for use on heavily exuding wounds, wounds prone to bleeding, fungating or infected wounds, sinus tracts and fistulas and may be left in place for up to seven days. They are not indicated for use on dry, black or necrotic wounds. They should be applied dry leaving a margin of at least 1 cm over the wound edges and secured with a secondary dressing (*Nurses' Index of Medicines and Products*, 2003).

Hydrogels

These are available in two amorphous formats: gels or a flat sheet. They have a high water content and do not swell in the wound like a hydrocolloid. They are suitable for desloughing and for light to medium exuding wounds and those wounds that are granulating. Sheet hydrogels do not require secondary dressings, whereas amorphous gels do. They may be used on infected wounds but not those where anaerobic infection is suspected. They are pain free to the patient on removal. Gels should be removed from the wound by irrigation with saline or water. If a sheet gel becomes dry when removal is due they too will require rehydration prior to removal (Stringfellow *et al.*, 2003).

Iodine-based wound dressings

These dressings have been used for the prevention of infection in superficial wounds. There are a variety of products available. However, iodine is rapidly deactivated in the presence of pus and as Leaper (1998) states, they may have a limited use as an anti-microbial. Iodine-based Cadexomer dressings have the ability to absorb the exudate in exchange for the iodine and allow for a slower release of iodine into the wound. Prior to using iodine-based products you must refer to the manufacturer's guidelines for the maximum number of dressings to be used for any one patient and also ensure that the patient does not have any allergies to iodine-based products.

Non-low adherent dressings

These dressings simply protect the wound by covering it. They have very little absorbency and as such are prone to leakage. They are also prone to sticking to the wound during removal, thus causing traumatic damage. They do not maintain a moist, warm, healing environment.

Silicone wound dressings

There are a variety of dressings under this heading. They are available as both a gel and sheet dressing. The gels help to flatten and soften scar tissue and may be used for several years after healing, to minimise scar formation. They are non-adherent and may be reused for the patient. Sheet dressings may be used on fragile and painful wounds with a secondary dressing to absorb exudate; they are useful in highly exuding wounds. You must check with the patient for any silicone allergies prior to application.

Semi-permeable film dressings

These are designed to protect the skin from the effects of moisture, friction and shear. They are resistant to urine and faeces and promote healing of excoriated skin. They should not be used on fragile or blistered skin and contain no absorbency properties. There are various products available in this category and you should read the application and removal instructions for each product prior to use. Care should be taken when removing the dressing to prevent damage to the good tissue and surrounding skin.

Silver dressings

These may be used on chronic ulcers and wounds colonised with bacteria, and are suitable for the treatment of partial and full thickness, moderately to heavily exuding wounds, but should be used with caution on patients with renal or hepatic disorders and should not be used on healthy skins as maceration may occur. The dressings must NOT be cut. Please refer to the manufacturer's guidelines prior to application.

Vacuum assisted closure®

Also known as the VAC®, this assists in the closure of wounds by applying localised negative pressure to draw the edges of the wound together. It creates a hypoxic environment within the wound bed in which anaerobic bacteria cannot survive. This environment forces the microcirculation to regenerate rapidly and produce large amounts of capillaries. At the same time the negative pressure will pull blood into the wound bed, bringing with it growth factors and macrophages to an area depleted by bacterial contamination. This leaves large reserves of oxygen for tissue regeneration (Miller & Glover, 1999).

The negative pressure also removes slough and loose necrotic material from the wound bed leaving it clean with an excellent blood supply, encouraging proliferation of granulation tissue and ensuring that white blood cells are supplied with oxygen through the bloodstream, while anaerobic bacteria in the wound bed die (Morykwas & Louis, 1993).

It may be used on chronic wounds, acute and traumatic wounds, meshed grafts, subacute wounds, partial thickness burns and open abdominal wounds. It should not be used on fistulas to organs or body cavities, necrotic tissue, untreated osteomyelitis, malignancy in the wound, or non-enteric fistulas where there is active bleeding, or patients with anti-coagulation disorders. You will need to take advice from the company's representatives regarding application and use of the system.

Wound drainage pouches

These dressings may be used as a primary or secondary dressing to cover an absorbent dressing and to collect large amounts of exudate. They are drained while leaving the pouch in situ and should be cut to shape to fit each individual wound (*Nurses' Index of Medicines and Products*, 2003).

Table 7.2 offers a review of the dressings we have discussed in this chapter.

Choosing the dressing

When choosing a wound dressing you should take into account the following:

- What does the wound need to ensure the correct environment is achieved?
- Is the dressing available in both the hospital and community?
- Is it cost effective? You will need to ask how often does the dressing require changing, as it is not just the cost of the dressing, but also the nursing time associated with the procedure.
- Are there independent product trials and literature available?
- Is the patient happy with your choice and do they understand how it works?
- Is the dressing easy to use?
- What do you want the dressing to achieve? That is to say, do you want it to manage fluid exudate, control odour or help to manage pain, etc?

Remember, the first dressing of choice may not be the final, because as the wound heals, dressings will change as appropriate to the stage of healing. Please refer to Box 7.2 for criteria for choosing a dressing. This will provide a checklist for you when choosing a dressing. In addition to these traditional dressings, there may be occasions when other techniques are necessary. These include: growth factors, tissue engineering, electrical stimulation, ultrasound, hydrotherapy and laser treatment.

Table 7.2 Overview of wound dressings and indications for their use.

Generic name of dressing	Indications for use
Alginates	Moderate to heavily exuding wounds. Do NOT use on dry wounds. Have haemostatic properties.
Biosurgey	Also known as larvae. Infected or necrotic wounds. Not be to used in a fistulae or wounds that may connect to vital organs.

Table 7.2 *Continued*

Generic name of dressing	Indications for use
Cadexomer bead	Moderately exuding wounds; infected, sloughy or chronic wounds. Do NOT use on dry wounds. Contain iodine, therefore check for any iodine sensitivities prior to use.
Foams	Most types of wounds from low to heavily exuding.
Hydrocolloids	Low to moderate exuding wounds. May be used for debriding dry to moist devitalised tissue.
Hydrofibre	Heavily exuding wounds or wounds that are bleeding, fungating or infected. Not for use on dry, black or necrotic wounds.
Hydrogels	Low to moderately exuding wounds. Rehydrate wounds. May be used for desloughing. Can be used on infected wounds but NOT with an anaerobic infection.
Non-low adherent	Dry to lightly exuding wounds. Not recommended for clinically infected words or wounds that are heavily exuding.
Iodine-based dressings	Aids in the prevention of infection. Contain iodine, therefore check the patient's sensitivities prior to application.
Semi-permeable dressings	To protect skin, e.g. reddened areas or on very lightly exuding wounds. Often used as a secondary dressing. Do NOT use on fragile skin.
Silicone gels	Recently healed wounds.
Silicone sheets	Highly exuding painful wounds.
Silver	Moderately to heavily exuding wounds. Chronic ulcers and wounds colonised with bacteria. Not for use on healthy skin due to the risk of maceration, or patients with renal or hepatic disorders. The dressing must NOT be cut.
Carbon	Odourous low exudate wounds.
Vacuum assisted closure	Closure of wounds. Not to be used on fistulae to organs or body cavities, necrotic tissue, untreated osteomyelitis, malignancy in the wound or non-enteric fistulae where there is active bleeding or on patients with anticoagulation disorders.
Wound drainage pouches	Primary or secondary dressings to collect large amounts of exudate.

Box 7.2 Criteria for choosing a dressing (Miller & Collier, 1996, p. 20).

(1) Choose a dressing that maintains a moist environment at the wound/dressing interface. The only possible exceptions are peripheral necrosis secondary to arterial disease and diabetic ulcers, where the risk of rapid infection may be increased by a wet environment.

(2) Choose a dressing that is able to control (remove) exudate. A moist wound environment is good; a wet environment is not beneficial.

(3) Choose a dressing that does not stick to the wound and cause trauma on removal.

(4) Choose a dressing that protects the wound from the outside environment.

(5) Choose a dressing that will aid debridement if there is sloughy or necrotic tissue in the wound.

(6) Choose a dressing that will keep the wound close to body temperature.

(7) Choose a dressing that is acceptable to the patient.

(8) Cost: if used properly modern wound care products will be cost effective.

(9) Availability, both in the hospital and community.

(10) Oxygen permeability.

(11) Wound pH.

(12) Particulate matter.

Reproduced with kind permission from the *Professional Nurse*, Emap Healthcare.

Dressing the wound

Now you have completed the assessment of the ulcer and chosen the most appropriate dressing it is time to apply the dressing to the ulcer/wound. You should collect all the equipment from the treatment room prior to going to the patient to undertake the procedure. This will prevent you having to go back and forth to collect equipment when you have reached the patient's bed area. When you reach the patient with your equipment it is imperative that you explain to the patient what you intend to do and gain their consent to treatment before you commence the procedure. When the patient has given their consent and they are happy for you to start the procedure then you must ensure privacy for the patient by drawing the curtains around the patient's bed. If there is a treatment room available, with an examination couch available, and the patient is fit to go to the treatment room, then this may be a more appropriate environment in which to carry out the dressing. You should wash your hands before opening all your equipment and following setting up of your equipment. If gloves are to be worn, hands should be washed prior to putting the gloves on. The procedure should be a clean technique and should follow your hospital's or employer's guidelines and recognised policy.

The first procedure that should be carried out is the removal of any dead or infected tissue, by a competent practitioner. You should cleanse the wound with warm normal saline if necessary. Bacteria often contaminate many pressure ulcers, but with no clinical signs of multiplication or host reaction. Therefore, it is unnecessary to swab these wounds unless there are signs of clinical infection (Gilchrist, 1994). He maintains that with wound infection topical antibiotics and other applications are inappropriate; only systemic antibiotics will be effective. Therefore, when you are applying your dressing you are maintaining a warm, moist environment and preventing further contamination. Box 7.3 identifies the clinical signs of wound infection.

Box 7.3 Clinical signs of wound infection.

- Localised heat
- Increased pain (at the wound site or surrounding skin)
- Increased exudate and discharge
- Cellulites
- Malodourous

Table 7.3 Most commonly used wound dressings.

Hydrocolloids: these dressings interact with the wound moisture and form a gel. They also possess occlusive properties and may be left in place for between 5–7 days.

Hydrogels: they come in two forms, either a sheet or a gel. The gels have high water content and should ideally be used on wounds that are already heavily exuding.

Film dressings: these are transparent and may be used on superficial wounds.

Alginates: these come in sheets and as a roll for cavities. They are for exuding and not dry wounds. You should not moisten them prior to application.

Foam dressings: these can contain large amounts of exudate and are available as sheets and cavity fillers. They can be adhesive or non-adhesive, so are useful for patients with friable skin.

Particulates: these are useful for infected wounds. They interact with moisture to form a gel or paste and are occlusive.

You should explain to the patient what you are doing and ensure that they are comfortable during the procedure. You should not be causing excessive pain to the patient. If the wound dressing is painful to remove or if the surrounding site is painful, then please remember to administer prescribed analgesia prior to commencing and allow enough time for the analgesia to take effect prior to performing the dressing change. If prescribed, entonox may be effective in relieving the patient's pain during the procedure. The wound dressing chosen must ensure that the optimum wound healing environment is maintained and this should be undertaken using a clean technique. As we have discussed earlier, there are a variety of wound dressing products for you to choose from. Table 7.3 highlights the ones that are most frequently used for the dressing of a pressure ulcer.

When you have completed the dressing change, the patient should be made comfortable, you should again wash your hands and dispose of the equipment as per your local policy. Sharps will need to be placed in the correct sharps container and any infected or soiled dressings should be placed in the appropriate bags for disposal. All equipment should be returned to the treatment room and not left at the bedside. When the procedure is complete you must document all your actions in the care plan.

CONCLUSION

You will have noted from this chapter that there are a variety of wound dressings to choose from. All the dressings will profess to heal wounds and the representatives will provide you with literature to support their claims. While many of these products have undergone trials on their performance you must always read the available literature and critically analyse its validity. Look at who wrote the articles and who undertook these trials: were they independent trials or did the companies perform the trials? The dressings that you use are medicines and it is vitally important that you understand the properties of these dressings and any contraindications for their use. If you do not understand how a specific dressing works, you must investigate and develop your knowledge prior to using it. Always inform the patient what the dressing is and why you have chosen that particular one. Always gain the patient's consent prior to using the dressing. You would not administer any medication if you did not understand what it was for, and therefore you must apply the same concepts to the administration of wound dressings. Company representatives will always be willing to advise you, as will your tissue viability specialist, or the tissue viability link nurse for your unit.

SELF-ASSESSMENT

After reading this chapter you should now take some time to reassess your knowledge base.

Reflection

Take some time to reflect upon the knowledge you have gained and how you will implement it into your own practice.

What knowledge did I possess prior to reading this chapter?

What do I know now?

How will my practice change as a result of attaining this knowledge?

Do I need to discuss with anyone practices I have witnessed that are not evidence-based, in relation to my new knowledge?

If so, who will I speak to?

Scenario

You are a third-year student nurse and have been asked by your mentor to assist her in a wound dressing of a 72-year-old man who has developed a grade four pressure ulcer, using the EPUAP grading system, to his sacrum. You remove a hydrocolloid wound dressing and discover that the wound is very wet in appearance, with green exudate, malodourous and the surrounding skin is becoming excoriated.

Tips on completing the scenario
Below is some information that you may have considered while working through the scenario. It is not an exhaustive list but it will give you some guidance on the information you should have collected.

You should have considered reassessing the wound, as it appears that it has deteriorated. As the wound is producing exudate that is green in colour, it suggests an infection. A wound swab will be required and consideration should be given to changing the dressing regime. You may want to consider using a silver based dressing, with carbon and a foam to aid in combating the infection and controlling the odour and exudate. Medical staff should be informed to allow for an assessment of the use of antibiotics. You may also want to refer the patient to the tissue viability specialist for expert advice. Documentation will need to include a reassessment of the wound and the surrounding skin, photograph, drawing or tracing of the wound (dependent on the local guidelines), pain assessment, and details of the wound swab and referrals to other members of the interdisciplinary team, as well as details of the new dressing regime. It is worth considering a nutritional assessment and referral to the dietician, as the wound is exudating heavily and vital nutrients will be being lost. In addition, the patient may be feeling unwell due to the infection, and may not feel like eating.

REFERENCES

Black, D. (1982) *Inequalities in Health* (Black Report) Penguin, Harmondsworth.

Department of Health (2001) *Essence of Care. Patient Focused Benchmarking for Healthcare Practitioners*. Department of Health, London.

EPUAP European Ulcer Advisory Panel (1999) Guidelines on treatment of pressure ulcers. *Epuap Review*, **1**, 7–8.

Flanagan, M. (1997) Wound cleansing. In: *Nursing Management of Chronic Wounds* (eds Morison, M., Moffatt, C., Bridel-Nixon, J. & Bale, S.), pp. 87–101. Mosby, London.

Flanagan, M. & Fletcher, J. (2003) Tissue viability: managing chronic wounds. In: *Nursing Adults: The Practice of Caring* (eds Brooker, C. & Nicol, M.), p. 183. Mosby. Elsevier Science Limited, London.

Gilchrist, B. (1994) Treating bacterial wound infection. *Nursing Times*, **90** (50), 55–8.

Leaper, D. (1998) Antiseptic toxicity in open wounds. *Nursing Times*, **84** (25), 77–9.

Miller, M. & Collier, M. (1996) Understanding wounds. *Professional Nurse*, p. 20. Macmillan Magazines, London.

Miller, M. & Glover, D. (1999) *Wound Management Theory and Practice*. Emap Healthcare Ltd, London.

Morison, M. & Moffatt, C. (1997) Leg ulcers. In: *A Colour Guide to the Nursing and Management of Chronic Wounds* (eds Morison, M., Moffatt, M., Bradel-Nixon, J. & Bale, S.). C. V. Mosby, London.

Morykwas, M. J. & Louis, C. (1993) Use of negative pressure to increase the rate of granulation tissue formation in chronic open wounds. *Proceedings of the Annual Meeting Federation of American Societies for Experimental Biology* (28 March–1 April). Federation of American Societies for Experimental Biology, New Orleans.

Nurses' Index of Medicines and Products (2003) 3rd edn. Mark Allen Group, Gwent.

Nursing and Midwifery Council (2002) *Code of Professional Conduct*. Nursing and Midwifery Council, London.

Ovington, L. (2001) Wound management: cleansing agents and dressings. In: *The Prevention and Treatment of Pressure Ulcers* (ed Morison, M. J.), pp. 135–54. Mosby, London.

Stringfellow, S., Russell, F., Cooper, P. J. & Gray, D. (2003) Wound care: accountability, consent and evidence. *The Nurses' Index of Medicines and Products 4*. pp. 202–17. (November). MA Healthcare Ltd, London.

Thomas, B. (1994) *Manual of Dietetic Practice*. 2nd edn. Blackwell Publishing, Oxford.

Williams, N. A. & Leaper, D. J. (1998) Infection. In: *Wounds: Biology and Management* (eds Leaper, D. J. & Harding, K. G.), pp. 71–8. Oxford Medical Publications, Oxford.

The Importance of Accurate Documentation, Legal, Ethical and Policy Issues

8

INTRODUCTION

Nurses rarely work in isolation and it is important to understand the context in which care takes place. The purpose of this chapter is to outline the policy, legal and ethical background to nursing care in relation to pressure areas, to emphasise the importance of accurate documentation. This chapter provides an introduction to this area of care by considering the background to policy development as well as a very brief discussion of selected UK health policies. We then go on to discuss legal and professional issues within nursing practice, before considering some of the principles applying to the ethics of nursing practice. Finally, we use the example of consent to treatment to draw together the key themes of the chapter.

LEARNING OBJECTIVES

By the end of this chapter the reader will be enabled to:

❑ Identify policy, legal and ethical issues relating to pressure areas
❑ Discuss the importance of accurate documentation
❑ Identify and discuss legal and professional issues
❑ Discuss ethical principles

Policy

Policy related to nursing moves at a rapid pace and the purpose of this section is to give you an insight into some of the contemporary issues in policy development. It is important for nurses to keep up-to-date with current policy because it has a profound effect on our working lives. The extent to which nurses are, or should, be involved with contributing to policy development is a debate that is explored elsewhere (Robinson, 1997). Our own view is that nurses, at the very least, have a responsibility to keep up-to-date with current issues and to recognise their own contribution to the implementation of current policy. Deborah Hennessy puts this well when she explains that whilst nurses should certainly be more involved in the development of health policy they are always involved in its implementation:

> 'Nurses know, recognise and meet patients' immediate health and social care needs. However, their patients' lives and their ability to be healthy are influenced by numerous policies affecting the environment within which they live, their lifestyles, public health needs and the health services available, as well as the nursing care provided'
>
> (Hennessy, 1999)

Nurses need to be aware of policies that affect their work, but it is also helpful to understand the reasons for the development of policy. This is particularly the case for those with an obvious attention to clinical work. *Essence of Care* (DoH, 2001) is a clear case in point. Government policy is designed to promote high standards of essential nursing care and developed from concerns that such care was poor in many areas. Similarly, clinical governance (DoH, 1997) was a policy that developed following a number of well publicised cases in which harm was caused to a number of patients following the perceived failure of professionals to understand the responsibility they had for their own actions.

Legal and professional issues

In addition to their obligations to their employers and their personal ethical code, nurses have two primary obligations in relation to their employment: one is to the law and the other is to their profession. Both provide a framework in which the nurse can practice safely, and both are designed to protect both practitioner and client.

The law

Law is made by a legislature (for example, Parliament in the UK and Congress in the USA) and is then interpreted and refined by the courts. Sometimes the courts go further than to interpret and refine existing laws when they have to make decisions about cases in which there is no legislation, as in the British cases of negligence. In Europe this fairly simple principle seems to have been complicated in recent years by the incorporation of some European legislation into national law. In the UK there are also two legal systems and parliaments, one for England, Wales and Northern Ireland and one in Scotland. The principle remains the same and it is important that nurses are aware of specific law within their own area. It is also important to remember that the law changes, either through new legislation or by further interpretation. A good example of this is the introduction of the Human Rights Act in the UK. This is an example of the UK Parliament incorporating a piece of European legislation into UK law. This has made a number of changes in the law of the UK, as the courts have had to make judgements on an increasing amount of cases that have been applied to the Human Rights Act.

There are two important points to bear in mind about the law: it is different in different countries and it constantly changes. Moreover, it is the responsibility of the individual to be aware of the law as it affects them; ignorance of the law is never accepted as an excuse in court.

Professional issues

There is a significant amount of published literature on professionalism and professionalisation. In short, the former discusses the responsibilities and behaviours expected of people in a professional position, while the latter explores the way in which professions have become important within society. This section will venture into both areas by trying to make sense of the importance of professional issues for nurses.

Professions are very different from each other and one of the main elements about nursing that sets it apart from other groups, including most of the other healthcare workers, is its sheer size. Nursing is easily the largest of the healthcare professions and this makes it intensely political. Decisions made about nursing tend to have important implications for health services and it is no coincidence that in most countries the process of nurse registration has been long fought and controversial. Unlike some other professions it is also noteworthy that governments always control a large element of the regulation of nursing. The extent of that control, however, varies from country to country and from period to period.

In professional terms there is a mandatory obligation to fulfil the clauses of the professional code of conduct. In the UK the code of conduct is written by the Nursing and Midwifery Council and other countries will have similar arrangements for their own professional code (ICN code).

Ethical issues

All nurses face ethical issues as part of their daily practice. Most such issues involve choices that may seem unimportant and about which decisions are often made rapidly by the nurse. Examples of this are the decision to prioritise areas of work, or the importance of the needs of more than one patient. Nurses are also faced with ethical issues when they decide whether to cut a conversation with a patient short or whether to inquire deeper into problems. They also have to make decisions about the information they pass on to colleagues or to relatives of a patient. Such decisions are part and parcel of nursing skills and are often the things that are remembered most by patients (either gratefully or resentfully). The commonplace nature of these issues makes them all the more important to consider within an ethical framework. Such a framework also encompasses the decisions about equally important, but often more newsworthy, choices about treatments. In these cases decisions are less likely to be left with one person and are often shared within a team of professionals working with the patient.

There are two principle elements to ethical care in nursing. First, the obligation to do good (sometimes referred to as beneficence) and second, to prevent harm (also referred to as non-maleficence).

Professional legal and ethical issues – duty of care

Our duty of care is a good example of an obligation that encompasses a legal, professional and moral obligation. As far as the law is concerned nurses are obliged among other things to:

- Fulfil the terms of their contract of employment
- Ensure that no act or omission might harm another (*Donaghue* v. *Stevenson*, 1932)
- Ensure that the standard of care is commensurate with a nurse who is the mirror image of you (*Bolam* v. *Friern Barnet HMC*, 1957)

This legal duty should always be considered within the context of current practice, particularly in relation to evidence-based practice, clinical governance, specialist and consultant nurses.

While few would doubt that nurses have a moral duty to care, there are different perspectives about what this means in both theory and in practice. For example, we cannot escape the fact that there are very different perspectives about issues such as abortion and euthanasia. Such debates often go to the heart of what is meant by personhood and the rights and obligations of individuals. Duties are owed to someone or something, perhaps in response to their right to expect something, or to serve their interests. For example, if we believe that people have a right to healthcare then someone has a duty to provide it. Alternatively, if we believe that as a society we have a duty to provide a system of healthcare then, although welfare might be maximised, individuals may not get what they consider their rights. This connects the moral duty to care to the political debates about the nature of healthcare that readers will be familiar with. The philosophical roots of the obligation to provide healthcare are fundamentally different for the individual, and also for political parties and movements. To help illuminate this we shall look very briefly at two philosophical perspectives within the context of the obligation to care.

Deontological perspectives

As a rational willing agent, you have a duty to act morally. This duty can be understood through practical reasoning, according to Kant (1964), using the categorical imperative. One should act as though one had a universal rule, for example, a duty to all. People should always be treated as an end in themselves, never as a means to the ends of others. An example of this is the view that the health service is for the benefit of service users not the service providers. The duty to care for patients may be greater because of the privileged relationship we share and the trust which patients place in their carers. Moral principles may help to further justify the duty of care but there are often conflicting duties.

For example, what is the nurse's duty of care to a 92-year-old woman who refuses to eat or drink and says she has had enough? There is a clear duty to respect her wishes, but also a duty to respect life itself. Even when this is tempered with the tenet 'thou needs not strive officiously to keep alive' the boundaries of one's duty remain hazy.

Utilitarian perspectives
The duty is to act in ways that maximise welfare, bringing about the greatest good for the greatest number of people. This has very clear consequences for individuals who may require expensive, time consuming or unusual treatments, because the resources required would be more effectively used if spread to many more people requiring less consuming treatment. On a national level, it could be argued that the welfare would be maximised if some services were allocated more resources, where others were reduced (this argument has justified the reduction in fertility services, for example).

Consent to treatment
Consent to treatment is a good example of the need to practice legally and ethically. Consent means to agree, comply with, acquiesce, authorise or permit. The only morally valid form of consent to treatment is informed consent. This is more than simply agreeing to a procedure, but means agreeing to something that is understood. Someone giving informed consent understands the nature of the procedure and its associated risks and benefits; they are aware of any alternatives and have had an opportunity to decline the treatment. No one can give consent to treatment on behalf of another adult. Exceptions to the general rule are very rare. In the case of incapacity, treatment can be carried out without consent and also if there is no one else legally competent to consent on the patient's behalf, providing that the treatment is necessary; it cannot be delayed until the patient is able to consent and is in the patient's best interests. Case law indicates that if the patient is incapable of giving valid consent a practitioner is acting lawfully provided that they follow approved practice and are acting in the best interests of the person (*F.* v. *West Berkshire Health Authority*, 1989).

For the vast majority of nursing procedures, therefore, informed consent is required and it is only in the most exceptional circumstances that it is not. Informed consent applies to the most simple, as well as the most complex of procedures and should never be assumed. If a patient is confused or has a learning disability you are still required morally and professionally to ensure that they give informed consent. In cases such as this it is important to remember that informed consent is not a single event and will need to be regularly visited.

Documentation

Good record keeping is a crucial element of nursing care for a number of reasons. It:

- Helps ensure continuity of care
- Aids assessment by recording changes
- Maintains a record of care for future reference

Accurate recording of patient care is an essential component of nursing. It is worth noting that there are several important principles that underpin this. All written records could be used for legal purposes at some stage and, should something go wrong, it may be several years before evidence is heard in court. It is useful to view record keeping as a process that can provide clear evidence of what was done, when, and by whom, as this can strengthen the case when high standards of care have been provided.

First, records should be legible and preferably written in black ink so that they may, if necessary, be copied for legal purposes. It is also important to sign and date each entry, as each nurse is accountable for the record they make. This is why student nurses should have their records countersigned by a registered nurse. Any deletions should be left visible and scored through with a single line. After all, you would not expect a bank to accept a cheque that had the amount covered with correction fluid! Records should be made as soon as possible after a particular episode of care.

Second, the language used needs to be considered. This should be professional, without using abbreviations or jargon that renders the text inaccessible to those outside the profession. The records should also avoid any judgemental comments and subjective material. This is particularly important where patients are partners in their care and discuss these with their carers, for example, in community practice. Increasingly, records are shared across a multidisciplinary team and clarity is of vital importance.

Lastly, the patient records need to be specific about care. In pressure area care this is crucial in order to monitor healing processes or deterioration of wounds. Such details could include size, depth and shape of the wound; types of wound care interventions, patient comfort and response to treatment and care.

Increasingly, nurses are recording care using electronic records. The principles are the same as for a paper-based system, although electronic records do present some different practical issues. The issue of confidentially, for example, is particularly important and local protocols need to include means of authenticating entries to records. The UK Access to Health Records Act (1990) enabled patients to see all written records about them made after 30 October 1991. This also applies to computer records and there are very few exceptions to this legal right. Nurses also need to be aware of the UK Data Protection Act (1984) that is designed to facilitate patient access to their records and stipulates how records should be stored and kept confidential.

Unfortunately this aspect of care is often overlooked when dealing with the most simple of procedures. This is in contrast to new or unusual procedures when there may be a degree of nervousness about consent, or subsequent disagreement. For example, the use of larval therapy is distasteful to many people and significant effort will be put into making sure patients understand and agree to treatment. In more conventional therapy such consent may be assumed rather than sought. Yet it is just as important in professional and ethical terms that informed consent is sought and recorded in order to protect from potential litigation.

CONCLUSION

This chapter has sought to introduce you to the policy, legal and ethical backgrounds to nursing care. It has necessarily only touched the surface of what is a complex area. We have separated the different elements of professional, legal and ethical aspects of nursing practice for the sake of clarity. The reality, however, is that in practice they need to be understood together because the position in most cases is that policy, the law and professional and ethical issues all have a substantial bearing. Whilst this is a complex area, most of the complexity is in the application as the principles are reasonably straight-forward and are fundamental to good nursing practice.

SELF-ASSESSMENT

After reading this chapter you should now take some time to reassess your knowledge base.

Reflection

Take some time to reflect upon the knowledge you have gained and how you will implement it into your own practice.

What knowledge did I possess prior to reading this chapter?

What do I know now?

How will my practice change as a result of attaining this knowledge?

Do I need to discuss with anyone practices I have witnessed that are not evidence-based, in relation to my new knowledge?

If so, who will I speak to?

Scenario

An 86-year-old gentleman is admitted to your ward. On admission he is frail and underweight. His family explain that he has been living with them for the last two months as his mental state has deteriorated and he has become very forgetful, leading him to forget when he has last eaten. On assessment of his pressure areas, you note that his bony prominences are red but there are no signs of broken skin.

Tips on completing the scenario

Below is some information that you may have considered while working through the scenario. It is not an exhaustive list but it will give you some guidance on the information you should have collected.

You will need to undertake various assessments on this gentleman that will include:

- Nutritional
- 'At risk'
- Moving and handling
- Pain

You will need to explain all procedures to him and obtain his consent prior to administering any interventions, for example, the use of a pressure redistributing device. Even though he is forgetful you will still need to obtain his consent. All interventions that you include in his care plan will require documenting and this will include details and results of the assessments you have used, dating his care plan and signing all entries. If you are unqualified this will require countersigning by a qualified practitioner.

You will also need to consider the moral and ethical principles of this gentleman's care if he does not understand the rationale for his care.

REFERENCES

Bolam v. Friern Barnet HMC (1957) All ER 118.

Department of Health (1997) *The New NHS: Modern and Dependable.* Cm 3807. The Stationery Office, London.

Department of Health (2001) *The Essence of Care: Patient Focused Benchmarking for Healthcare Professionals.* HMSO, London.

Donaghue v. Stevenson (1932) AC 562.

F. v. West Berkshire Health Authority (1989) All ER 545.

Hennessy, D. & Spurgeon, P. (eds) (1999). *Health Policy and Nursing, Influence, Development and Impact.* Macmillan Press, London.

ICN Code of Ethics for Nurses. International Council of Nurses. www.icn.ch/icncode.pdf

Kant, I. (1964) *Groundwork of the Metaphysics of Morals,* (translated by Paton, H.J.) Harper & Row, New York.

Robinson, J. (1997) Power, politics and policy analysis in nursing. In: *Nursing: a Knowledge Base for Practice.* A. Perry. Arnold, London.

The Role of the Interdisciplinary Team in Pressure Area Care

9

LEARNING OBJECTIVES

By the end of this chapter the reader will be enabled to:

❏ Identify members of the interdisciplinary team
❏ Discuss the roles of the members of the interdisciplinary team in relation to pressure area care
❏ Identify relevant policy issues

INTRODUCTION

In April 2001 the National Institute for Clinical Excellence published clinical guidance on pressure ulcer risk assessment and prevention. This document included a statement under the heading of education and training, stating: 'an interdisciplinary approach to the training and education of healthcare professionals should be adopted' (NICE, 2001, p. 4). Surprisingly, this document was written in 2001, yet Torrance (1983) had previously highlighted that the development of pressure ulcers was not an entirely new problem facing health professionals, but a constant problem that afflicts the debilitated, disabled and chronically ill.

Historically, pressure ulcers are not new phenomena to the field of health. From recordings as far back as the prophet Isaiah in the eighth century BC there have been references to the development of these debilitating wounds (Dealey, 1994).

Yet one may wonder how it has taken until 2001 to realise that an interdisciplinary approach to the prevention and treatment of these ulcers is considered best practice. Traditionally, the development of pressure ulcers was seen as a result of poor nursing care and not the multifaceted aetiology that is discussed today (Simpson *et al.* 1996). Florence Nightingale (1861) documented that pressure ulcers were due to the short-comings of the nurse and not the disease. Writings like this led to Charcot (1877), an eminent French doctor, to believe that doctors could do nothing about the prevention and treatment of these ulcers, and therefore they became a nursing problem, which also carried a burden of guilt with it if a pressure ulcer did develop (Dealey, 1992).

Another issue was that pressure ulcers were considered to be an exclusive problem of the elderly (Young & Dobrzanski, 1992). It is believed that 70% of all pressure ulcers occur in patients over the age of 70 (Young & Dobrzanski, 1992). Yet prevalence studies have identified younger patients at risk (Bliss, 1988), particularly those who have survived major illnesses, but have lasting disabilities (Hillan *et al.* 1997). These two previously held beliefs, that pressure ulcers were a nursing problem and that most patients who developed them were elderly, were central to a failure in an understanding of this complex problem and led to the lack of a multidisciplinary team approach to their management (Simpson *et al.* 1996).

Today, the issue about the ownership of pressure ulcer prevention and treatment is changing (Sutton & Wallace, 1990). Documents such as the *Pressure Ulcer Risk Assessment and Prevention* guidelines (Rycroft-Malone & McInness, 2000; NICE, 2001) and annual conferences, for example, the European Pressure Ulcer Advisory Panel Open meeting and Wounds UK, promote the complexity of these wounds and the need to work as a team to aid their prevention and treatment. As stated by the King's Fund Centre (1989) a pressure ulcer prevention policy requires a well planned strategy that brings into line current research and best practice, not an inconsistent and incoherent approach.

Not only is it imperative that nurses, doctors and professionals allied to medicine work together to prevent and treat pressure ulcers, it is equally important to work across the primary, secondary and tertiary boundaries (Bellingham & Stephens, 1999).

This requires effective and open communication from staff at the three levels of healthcare provision:

(1) Primary health care, for example, district nurses, general practitioners and community physiotherapists
(2) Secondary care within a hospital setting
(3) Tertiary care, where rehabilitation, respite or hospice care is required

Hibbs (1988) and Waterlow (1988) wrote that most pressure sores are preventable, at least 95%, and if a multidisciplinary team were to share the responsibility of this multifaceted problem, this would ensure cost effective prevention and treatment strategies to target effective resources (Simpson *et al.* 1996).

Multidisciplinary team roles

A quote by Torrance (1983, p. 72) describes how a team effort can promote success in the prevention and management of pressure ulcers:

'The nurses' turning schedule may be ineffective if systemic disease is not treated, while the wound care programme can be undermined if the patients' nutritional status is impaired. Even appropriate management of a pressure sore can be ineffective if the patient is apathetic and lacks motivation.'

Therefore, it is important to look at the different members of the multidisciplinary team and how their actions can have an effect on pressure ulcer prevention and management (Simpson *et al.* 1996).

Tissue viability nurse specialist

The emergence of this nurse specialist role came about because of a heightened awareness by purchasers and providers of the significant costs accrued by managing wounds incorrectly (Flanagan, 1996). The attributes the purchasers and providers expect this type of nurse to hold are: specialist skills within this complex field, the capability to manage change and advanced interpersonal skills (Flanagan, 1996). The purpose of this role is to take a lead in pressure ulcer prevention and management and work alongside other members of the multi-disciplinary team (James, 1994). By carrying out the four main roles of a nurse specialist position: nurse educator, nurse consultant, nurse manager and nurse researcher (James, 1994), the tissue viability nurse is in an ideal position to collaborate with all health professionals to bring about best practice and a true multidisciplinary approach (Bale, 1995).

The role of nurse consultant allows tissue viability nurses to make themselves available for specialist advice and/or consultation for patients whose wounds have not responded to first line policy, or where first line policy is not appropriate (Hamric & Spross, 1983). The nurse specialist may see a patient with a chronic pressure ulcer only once, or more regularly through follow up. Any assessment is always carried out in collaboration with other members of the multidisciplinary team, for example, district nurse, named nurse, or physician (Flanagan, 1992).

As a nurse educator, the tissue viability nurse provides up-to-date and evidence-based education and training to all members of the multidisciplinary team, ensuring that the level and type of information is specific to the group of healthcare staff being taught. Policies and procedures form a fundamental part of educational process and allow dissemination of specialist practice (James, 1994). Obviously these are written by a wound care advisory team, representing all the professionals who deal with patients at risk of, or who have, pressure ulcers (Hillan *et al.* 1997). Another aspect of the educational part of this role is to ensure adequate patient and carer information (NICE, 2001). The tissue viability nurse ensures that patients and carers are informed and educated about risk assessment and courses of action (NICE, 2001), and may even develop patient information leaflets with a wound care advisory group.

As all hospital expenditure has to be planned and monitored according to need, the tissue viability nurse has the important role of managing or negotiating with managers, budgets for the hire and purchase of pressure relieving/reducing equipment and wound dressings (Flanagan, 1996). Specialist knowledge in activity levels, preparing bids, current evidence-based practice and best buy can assist in achieving cost effective practice (Flanagan, 1992).

A nurse researcher also critically analyses the evidence provided by manufacturers, scientists, other nurse researchers, etc. within the field of pressure ulcer management. The development of policies and procedures is impacted by current research and this should also reflect education and training (James, 1994). The research aspect of the role also entails carrying out research and the auditing and monitoring of prevalence and incidence of pressure ulcers, product usage and pressure ulcer documentation (Flanagan, 1996). This information is then disseminated to other members of the multidisciplinary team via board meetings, education, training, etc.

Finally, the most important role of the tissue viability nurse as noted by James (1994, p. 61) is that: 'the nurse specialist can work with many groups of workers to ensure that all points in the patient's pathway promote tissue integrity'.

Directorate manager, hospital director and professional lead

Managers and directors have, in general, ultimate responsibility for the implementation and management of patient care (Simpson *et al.* 1996). They are required to do this through the allocation of resources and provision of educational support for their staff. They ensure suitable systems are in place to provide good quality pressure sore prevention. For example, they may ask for a report to be presented at executive level on an audit of the prevalence/incidence of pressure sores, equipment usage and correct product choice. They would then ascertain whether expenditure would need to increase or decrease on the purchase of equipment and educational input and make recommendations to the service.

Accountant

Trust accountants are an unusual consideration in the multi-disciplinary team. Yet to ensure the good management of equipment, dressings or staff required for pressure ulcer prevention and treatment one requires: 'good bookkeeping, financial planning and forecasting, negotiating with suppliers and treasurers and generating income skills' (Gebhardt, 1997, p. 91).

Doctor

According to Young and Roper (1996) doctors should have fundamental knowledge about pressure ulcer prevention and treatment, as they suggest that there will always be patients in any clinical speciality who have, or are at risk of, developing pressure ulcers. As medical staff have complete overall responsibility for patients' care (Simpson et al. 1996) and one of the possible complications of acute illness is pressure ulcer development (Bliss, 1988), it is essential that doctors from any speciality pay attention to vulnerable patients (Young & Roper, 1996).

It is widely thought that doctors should address issues such as: 'hydration, nutrition, respiratory function, circulation and infection, during treatment' (Simpson et al. 1996, p. 15; Young & Roper, 1996, p. 18) to aid prevention and treatment of these debilitating wounds. Medical staff carry out thorough assessments of their patients, as well as taking vital signs, bloods and other investigations. They are therefore in an ideal position to make early decisions on treatment (Browning, 1997), for example, commencing an intravenous infusion for a patient with sunken eyeballs and reduced skin turgor (Young & Roper, 1996) and rapid referrals to other members of the multidisciplinary team (Simpson *et al.* 1996), for example, to the dietician for a patient whose body mass index is under 20 and who has an albumin of 28.

Medication should be reviewed to see if the effect of sedatives or pain relief is reducing mobility as well as relieving the pain, as Exton-Smith (1961) highlighted the importance of spontaneous bodily movements reducing the incidence of pressure ulcer development. Other medication, such as antibiotics, may cause diarrhoea and increase the risk of excoriation and maceration of the skin (Dealey, 1994).

Other issues that could be addressed more proficiently, if medical staff became more involved in pressure ulcer management, would be the early treatment of wound infections and recognition of the quite distinct difference between liquefying necrosis and infection (Young & Roper, 1996). Improved wound management would occur, as knowledge of the main classes of wound care products would ensure accurate prescribing of appropriate products (Young & Roper, 1996) and the rapid referral to other disciplines such as the plastic surgeon, the general surgeon, or vascular surgeon for further advice and treatment (Browning, 1997).

Medical staff should also keep their patients and carers abreast of the current pressure ulcer management treatments, as well as the members of the multidisciplinary team who they may come into contact with. This ensures informed consent to treatment and reassures the patient that the team is working together for their best interests (Joffe *et al.* 2003). Medical staff are in an ideal position to aid multidisciplinary working within the field of pressure ulcer management as their high level of knowledge of the disease process and the subsequent effect on tissue integrity should alert them to initiating or referring those at risk to appropriate members of the multi-disciplinary team to improve patient outcomes (Rodeheaver *et al.* 1994).

Nurse

The Department of Health (2000b) states that the condition of registration is the ability of a nurse to be able to:

'undertake and document a comprehensive, systematic and accurate nursing assessment of the physical, psychological, social and spiritual needs of patients, clients and communities.

Provide a rationale for the nursing care delivered, which takes into account social, cultural, spiritual, legal, political and economic influences.

Evaluate and document the outcomes of nursing and other interventions'.

Therefore it is quite clear that nurses are in an ideal position to ensure the holistic management of patient care (Simpson *et al.* 1996).

When a patient is initially assessed, be it in hospital, at home, or in a hospice or nursing home, the registered nurse (this may be adult, mental health, or child nurse, midwife or health visitor) can quickly identify those patients at risk of pressure ulcer development, or who have existing skin damage (Rycroft-Malone & McInnes, 2000). Reassessment is then compared to the initial assessment and any changes in the patient's condition noted (NICE, 2001).

A plan of care is implemented and evaluated, based on appropriate evidence-based practice (DoH, 2000a). Patients found to be at risk, or who have ulcers, should be supplied with a suitable mattress and cushions, (*Effective Health Care Bulletin*, 1995) with the equipment checked to see if it is in good working order (Simpson *et al.* 1996). The registered nurse also regularly reassesses the appropriateness of the equipment for the risk level of their patient.

If a piece of equipment requires servicing, or is found to be faulty, then the registered nurse should report the fault to the company who tends to the mattress contract or the central agent who deals with servicing and maintenance of equipment within the organisation, for example, the bioengineers or estates department (Glenister, 2000). As registered nurses are accountable for the nursing care a patient may receive they should also ensure that any healthcare support workers or student nurses who are assisting with pressure ulcer management are adequately supervised (NMC, 2002). Registered nurses should also refer to other health professionals or seek guidance when they are aware that their knowledge is inadequate, in order to find solutions to their patients' problems (NMC, 2002), for example, the tissue viability nurse when they have exhausted first line policy, the dietician regarding supplemental feeding, the doctor for further investigations or prescription of medications (Franks, 1999). Some qualified nurses may choose to become a tissue viability link nurse, who acts as a link between the tissue viability nurse and staff on their ward, unit, practice or home.

This system provides a close association with staff and patients and avoids fragmentation of care (Hamric & Spross, 1983). The purpose of such a service is for the tissue viability nurse to disseminate their knowledge to the link nurses and provide support, advice and education on the aetiology of pressure ulcers, the preventative and treatment methods and appropriate usage of equipment and dressings (Franks, 1999). As the link nurse's knowledge and skills develop within the field of pressure sore management, the staff within his/her clinical field can utilise him/her as the first point of contact when a patient's care does not match policy and procedure. They can also disseminate any new knowledge and skills they have learnt from the tissue viability nurse meetings to other members of staff and educate students, healthcare assistants, patients and carers (Simpson *et al.* 1996). Not only should this link nurse service be open to nurses but also to other healthcare professionals who are enthusiasts within the system, for example, occupational therapists and physiotherapists.

Healthcare assistant

The role of a healthcare assistant in pressure ulcer management is to support the registered nurse in the delivery of care (RCN, 1993). They have the responsibility to ensure that specific aspects of patient care are instigated, for example, the feeding of patients and recording of food and drink consumption, to ensure adequate nutritional intake; the turning of patients who are immobile, based upon an individual patient turning regime. The healthcare assistant also has the responsibility of disclosing any changes in the patient's condition and skin integrity (Simpson *et al.* 1996).

Dietician

Dieticians have indepth knowledge of the importance of detailed nutritional and hydrational assessment and are able to provide advice and plan appropriate dietary requirements (Simpson *et al.* 1996), as severe protein malnutrition is linked with the development of pressure ulcers (Cullum & Clark, 1992) and failure of wounds to heal (Goode, 1990). Registered nurses should generally initiate nutritional assessment, for example, recording and taking into consideration diseases affecting nutritional intake, fluid balance charting, food diaries, assistance with feeding, and body mass index. Then, on the evaluation of these systems, they may seek further advice from a dietician (Hogston & Simpson, 2002). Once the dietician has assessed the patient they will make recommendations for types of feeding, supplements or snacks and will also follow up the patient, monitoring their progress.

Physiotherapist

Physiotherapists are equally as important to the multidisciplinary team, as their role in the prevention and treatment of pressure ulcers is twofold (Simpson *et al.* 1996).

Physiotherapists encourage independence and enhance voluntary movement with the use of physical methods, with the aid of heat, light, massage, manipulation and remedial exercise (McFerran, 1998). They can also teach other professionals how to handle and position patients to improve posture and body alignment, but also to reduce the risk of tissue damage (Simpson *et al.* 1996). These two roles assist in reducing the effects of pressure, shear and friction (Morison *et al.* 1997).

Occupational therapist

The role of the occupational therapist is to assess and maximise a patient's functional abilities and promote independence (McFerran, 1998). After an initial assessment, the occupational therapist discusses with the multidisciplinary team and the patient any problems that were noticed at assessment. They will then make recommendations for equipment to be used to reduce the risk of pressure ulcer damage, for example, cushions, seating, wheelchairs, banana boards (Browning, 1997). Each patient is followed up on regular occasions to re-evaluate their progress, to readapt and modify pressure relieving/reducing devices and check suitability for the present or other pieces of equipment (Simpson *et al.* 1996). The occupational therapist is extremely important to the prevention and management of pressure ulcers, as many patients with severe disabilities require custom made equipment to prevent or treat pressure ulcers. The equipment should also benefit the user by improving their quality of life and allow a patient to continue to pursue activities at home, and also at work (Browning, 1997).

Rehabilitation engineer

The purpose of this health professional's role within pressure ulcer management is to consider the risk/cause of pressure ulcer damage in wheelchair users and to determine and oversee pressure ulcer problems (Browning, 1997). The engineer also supplies pressure reducing/relieving equipment and discusses with patients and carers their role in prevention and management.

Plaster technician

Ill-fitting plastercasts and splints can increase the risk of pressure damage on an already susceptible limb. Therefore, a plaster technician can reduce the risk by appropriate fitting and designing of protective casts, not only to immobilise or support the affected limb, but to reduce the pressure applied to the skin (Browning, 1997). These casts can be made of lightweight material, which can aid mobility for a patient and reduce the risk of pressure elsewhere, for example, on the sacrum/buttocks from increased sitting.

Orthotist/prosthetist

According to NHS Careers (2003) a prosthetist ensures that the most appropriate artificial limb is fitted and made for a patient who was either born without a limb or who has lost a limb. An orthotist, however, supplies suitable aids such a splints, footwear and braces to relieve pressure, improve movement and remedy alignment (International Working Group on the Diabetic Foot, 1999). Their roles in relation to pressure ulcer development are to provide relief by ensuring a correctly fitted prosthetic limb or splint does not apply significant enough pressure to cause damage, but actually improves the mobility of a patient without compromising tissue integrity.

Product evaluation nurse

As pressure reducing and relieving equipment and dressings are used every day by most healthcare professionals, it is important that they are safe to use, are used correctly and are the best available in relation to cost, quality and evidence (Glenister, 2000). A product evaluation nurse has a responsibility to assist in quality trials and evaluations of the latest pressure reducing/relieving equipment for the prevention and treatment of pressure ulcers (Stephens, 2001).

Podiatrist

Many diabetic foot ulcers are due to ill-fitting shoes (Morison *et al.* 1997) or abnormal foot pressures (International Working Group on the Diabetic Foot, 1999), causing pressure to the skin with the added complication of friction. Underlying neuropathy and vascular insufficiency further increase the possibility of tissue breakdown (Dealey, 1994) and therefore, the patient requires regular review by the podiatrist. If a diabetic foot ulcer goes untreated or is not reviewed by the diabetic foot team, then it can have serious consequences, for example, sepsis and amputation (International Working Group on the Diabetic Foot, 1999). Diabetic foot patients should be under the care of a podiatrist to tend to their toenails and to check their feet regularly. Rapid referrals should be made to the podiatrist if any callus formation, lesions and ulcers develop.

Other nurse specialists

As friction and shear are often associated with poor moving and handling techniques (Berlowitz, 1989), it is imperative that correct procedures are performed (RCN, 2003). The back care coordinator is a specialist nurse whose responsibilities are to ensure approved education and training of both staff and patients and the appropriate purchase and usage of equipment to aid handling of patients and reduce the risk of back injuries.

Jordan and Clark (1977) found, during a pressure ulcer prevalence study, that 15.5% of those with ulcers were incontinent of urine and 39.7% were faecally incontinent. Although it is important to clean patients who have been incontinent, constant washing dries the skin by removing naturally occurring body oils (Dealey, 1994). Factors causing the incontinence and further aggravating the skin problem should be explored. If further advice is required a continence advisor can assist in the appropriate choice of incontinence aids, skin cleansers and barrier creams (Browning, 1997).

The general poor health of a patient is a contributory factor towards the development of pressure ulcers, for example, cardiac problems (Dealey, 1994), shock (Barton, 1977), peripheral vascular disease (Simpson *et al.* 1996) and diabetes (International Working Group on the Diabetic Foot, 1999). If a patient requires more information and support than the ward, clinic or nursing home staff can provide then referral to the cardiac nurse, the vascular nurse specialist and the diabetes nurse specialist is appropriate. They can advise on suitable management of the patient's condition and reduce the effects on tissue integrity.

Radiographers/radiologists

As many patients who attend radiography departments are attending for X-rays, scans, treatments and imaging, it is important that radiographers and radiologists have an appreciation of the cause of pressure sores, as many patients may have to lie in one position for long periods of time, increasing the risk of pressure ulcer development (Brown, 2002). There should be regular monitoring of the tables and trolleys used to ensure they are of adequate thickness to reduce the pressure on the skin and take into consideration the risk status of the patient (Brown, 2002).

Porters

Porters are an essential part of the multidisciplinary team as they transfer patients from one clinical area to another. Their role in relation to pressure ulcer prevention and management is to ensure patients are transferred in a suitable and prompt manner (Simpson *et al.* 1996). It is also important that if they are responsible for the delivery and removal of specialist pressure reducing and relieving equipment they protect the equipment from harm and store it correctly and safely (Glenister, 2000).

Bioengineers and estates departments

Depending on the trust in which one works the maintenance and performance of equipment should be managed within the controls assurance programme (NHS Executive, 1999) by a bioengineering or estates department. The equipment should be cleaned, serviced and maintained in compliance with guidance from the Medical Devices Agency (1998). This will ensure that all pressure reducing and relieving equipment used is safe and appropriate to prevent and treat pressure ulcers.

Equipment suppliers

There are many ways of acquiring equipment from commercial companies. This could be direct purchase, loan or contract. It is imperative, however, before giving a company responsibility for the supply of equipment, be it dressings or mattresses etc., that the suppliers agree to prompt attention to orders and goods delivered on time (Simpson *et al.* 1996). It is important, within the field of pressure ulcer prevention and treatment, that mattresses are used appropriately and promptly, as pressure of high levels for short periods of time and low pressures for long periods of time are detrimental to the skin (Reswick, 1976). This is due to the intensity and duration (Brand, 1976).

Patients and carers

NICE (2001, p. 5) suggest: 'patients who are able and willing should be informed and educated about risk assessment and resulting prevention strategies. This strategy should, where appropriate, include carers'. The document also includes a patient information leaflet that includes the heading 'working together' (p. 10). According to Watkinson (2002) nursing practice includes assisting patients to attain improved health. At all levels, primary, secondary and tertiary, each nurse can critically assess the situation and review how they can have an impact on health improvement. Within the field of pressure ulcer management it is as equally important for patients and carers to contribute to the multidisciplinary team effort as the other health professionals involved. It is clearly quite difficult to plan care for a patient without their involvement (Benbow, 1996), but apparently it still does happen (Joffe *et al.* 2003).

Patients are responsible for their own health gains (Watkinson, 2002) and should try to avoid damaging their health, by reducing risks (Simpson *et al.* 1996). Yet most patients require information on the risks of pressure ulcer development and treatment and therefore require extra input from the multidisciplinary team (Benbow, 1996). This effort to try and avoid pressure ulcers through effective education and support involves active participation and decision making (Benbow, 1996).

CONCLUSION

It is generally considered that pressure ulcers are preventable (EHCB, 1995), yet they account for 4–10% of patients admitted into hospital (Clark & Watts, 1994); the financial costs to the NHS are considerable (Cullum *et al.* 1995). Pressure ulcers are not a new phenomenon (Torrance, 1983) and over the last decade many worthy initiatives have been published to try and address the problem (DoH 1992, 1993, 2000*a*; Rycroft-Malone & McInness, 2000; NICE, 2001). Each of these documents discusses multidisciplinary working as the main contributing factor to reduce this problem and if members of the multidisciplinary team embrace their roles and develop an informed and dynamic attitude to prevention, the problem may be defeated and confined (Torrance, 1983).

SELF-ASSESSMENT

After reading this chapter you should now take some time to reassess your knowledge base.

Reflection

Take some time to reflect upon the knowledge you have gained and how you will implement it into your own practice.

What knowledge did I possess prior to reading this chapter?

What do I know now?

How will my practice change as a result of attaining this knowledge?

Do I need to discuss with anyone practices I have witnessed that are not evidence-based, in relation to my new knowledge?

If so, who will I speak to?

Scenario

Mrs Jones, a 27-year-old paraplegic lady, is due for discharge home in one week's time. She has an established grade 3 pressure ulcer to her sacrum that had developed prior to admission. She wishes to be discharged home, as it is her daughter's sixth birthday next week.

Tips on completing the scenario
Below is some information that you may have considered while working through the scenario. It is not an exhaustive list but it will give you some guidance on the information you should have collected.

Use of moving and handling, 'at risk' and wound grading assessment tools will require consideration. Involvement of community services will need examining, for example, the district nursing team, community occupational therapist and physiotherapist. You may also have assessed Mrs Jones for social service input and extra financial help if she is not claiming all the benefits she is entitled to. A wound dressing regime will need to be developed, with evidence to support its effectiveness, and reassessment dates. Adaptations in the home may be required, for example, pressure redistributing aids on discharge. These adaptations will need to be implemented prior to discharge home and will require assessment by the occupational therapists, physiotherapists and district nurses.

REFERENCES

Bale, S. (1995) The role of CNS within the healthcare team. *Journal of Wound Care*, **4** (2), 86–7.

Barton, A. (1977) Prevention of pressure sores. *Nursing Times*, **73** (41), 1593–5.

Bellingham, J. & Stephens, M. (1999) Bridging the hospital-community gap. *Community Nurse*, **5** (8), 51–2.

Benbow, M. (1996) Pressure sore guidelines: patient/carer involvement and education. *British Journal of Nursing*, **5** (3), 182–7.

Berlowitz, D. R. (1989) Risk factors for pressure sores: a comparison of cross-sectional and cohort derived data. *Journal of American Geriatrics Society*, **37**, 1043–50.

Bliss, M. R. (1988) Prevention and management of pressure sores. *Update*, 1 May, (36), 2258–67.

Brand, P. W. (1976) Pressure sores – the problem. In: *Bed Sore Biomechanics* (eds Kenedi, R. M., Cowden, J. M. & Scales, J. T.), University Park Press, Baltimore.

Brown, A. (2002) Pressure ulcer prevention in X-ray departments. Sixth European Pressure Ulcer Panel Open Meeting. Budapest, Hungary.

Browning, D. (1997) A team approach to pressure relief for people with disabilities. *Journal of Wound Care*, **6** (6), 298–300.

Charcot, J. M. (1877) *On Diseases of the Nervous System.* New Sydenham Society, Philadelphia.

Clark, M. & Watts, S. (1994) The incidence of pressure sores in a National Health Service Trust hospital during 1991. *Journal of Advanced Nursing*, **20**, 33–6.

Cullum, N. & Clark, M. (1992) Intrinsic factors associated with pressure sores in elderly people. *Journal of Advanced Nursing*, **17**, 427–31.

Cullum, N., Deeks, J. J. & Fletcher, A. W. (1995) Preventing and treating pressure sores. *Quality in Health Care*, **4**, 289–97.

Dealey, C. (1992) Pressure sores: the result of bad nursing? *British Journal of Nursing*, **1** (15), 748.

Dealey, C. (1994) *The Care of Wounds*. Blackwell, London.

Department of Health (1992) *The Health of the Nation. A Strategy for Health in England*. HMSO, London.

Department of Health (1993) *Pressure Sores: a Key Quality Indicator*. HMSO, London.

Department of Health (2000*a*) *Benchmarking the Fundamental Aspects of Care*. HMSO, London.

Department of Health (2000*b*) *Nurses Midwives and Health Visitors (Training) Amendment rules approval order*. HMSO, London.

Effective Health Care Bulletin (1995) *Effective Healthcare: the Prevention and Treatment of Pressure Sores*, **2** (1), 1–16.

European Pressure Ulcer Advisory Panel: www.epuap.org

Exton-Smith, A. N. (1961) The prevention of pressure sores: the significance of spontaneous bodily movements. *Lancet*, **2**, 1124–6.

Flanagan, M. (1992) The role of the nurse specialist in wound care. *Journal of Wound Care*, **1** (2), 45–6.

Flanagan, M. (1996) A contemporary approach to wound care education. *Journal of Wound Care*, **4** (9), 422–4.

Franks, Y. (1999) Healthy alliances in wound management. *Journal of Wound Care*, **8** (1), 13–17.

Gebhardt, K. S. (1997) Professional roles – the role of the clinical nurse specialist in pressure sore prevention (CNS-PSP). *Journal of Tissue Viability*, **7** (3), 51–4.

Glenister, H. (2000) The importance of using medical devices correctly. *Professional Nurse*, **16** (2), 905–8.

Goode, A. W. (1990) The metabolic basis of wound healing. In: *Pressure Sores: Clinical Practice and Scientific Approach* (ed. Bader, D. L.). Macmillan, London.

Hamric, A. B. & Spross, J. A. (1983) *The Clinical Nurse Specialist in Theory and Practice*. Grune and Stratton, New York.

Hibbs, P. (1988) *Pressure Area Care Policy*. City of Hackney Health Authority, London.

Hillan, E. M., Smith, L. N., Swaffield, J., Fraser, A. K. & Durie, M. (1997) *The Prevention and Management of Pressure Sores: a Multidisciplinary Approach to Audit*. University of Glasgow, Glasgow.

Hogston, R. & Simpson, P. M. (2002) *Foundations of Nursing Practice: Making the difference*. Palgrave Macmillan, Basingstoke.

International Working Group on the Diabetic Foot (1999) *International Consensus on the Diabetic Foot*. International Working Group on the Diabetic Foot, Amsterdam.

James, H. (1994) Exploring the role of the tissue viability specialist nurse. *Nursing Standard*, **9** (6), 60–3.

Joffe, S., Manocchia, M., Weeks, J. C. & Cleary, P. D. (2003) What do patients value in their hospital care? An empirical perspective on autonomy centred bioethics. *Journal of Medical Ethics*, **29**, 103–8.

Jordan, M. M. & Clark, M. (1977) *Report on Incidence of Pressure Sores in the Patient Community of the Greater Glasgow Health Board Area*. University of Strathclyde, Glasgow.

King's Fund Centre (1989) *The Prevention and Management of Pressure Sores within Health Districts*. King's Fund Centre for Health Services Development, London.

McFerran, T. A. (ed.) (1998) *Oxford Mini Dictionary for Nurses*. 4th edn. Oxford University Press, Oxford.

Medical Devices Agency (1998) *Medical Device and Equipment Management for Hospital and Community Based Organisations*. MDA DB9801. Department of Health, London.

Morison, M., Moffat, M., Bradel-Nixon, J. & Bale, S. (1997) *Nursing Management of Chronic Wounds*. Mosby, London.

National Health Service Careers (2003) Allied health professionals: What does a prosthetist and orthotist do? http://www.nhscareers.nhs.uk/nhs-knowledge_base/data/4908.html Accessed 7 August 2003.

National Health Service Executive (1999) *Controls Assurance Standard: Medical Devices Management*. Department of Health, London.

National Institute for Clinical Excellence (2001) *Pressure Ulcer Risk Assessment and Prevention*. NICE, London.

Nightingale, F. (1861) *Notes on Nursing*. Appleton Century, New York.

Nursing and Midwifery Council (2002) *Code of Professional Conduct*. Nursing and Midwifery Council, London.

Reswick, J. B. (1976) Experience at Ranchos Los Amigos Hospital with devices and techniques to prevent pressure sores. In: *Bedsore Biomechanics* (eds Kennedy, R. M., Cowden, J. M. & Scales, J. T.) University Park Press, Baltimore.

Rodeheaver, G., Baharestani, M. M., Brabec, M. E., *et al*. (1994) Wound healing and wound management: focus on debridement. *Advances in Wound Care*, **7** (1), 22–6.

Royal College of Nursing (1993) *The Role of the Support Worker within the Professional Nursing Team*. Royal College of Nursing, London.

Royal College of Nursing (2003) *Safer Staff Better Care: RCN Manual Handling, Training Guidance and Competencies*. Royal College of Nursing, London.

Rycroft-Malone, J. & McInnes, E. (2000) *Pressure Ulcer Risk Assessment and Prevention*. Technical Report. Royal College of Nursing, London.

Simpson, A., Bowers, K. & Weir-Hughes, D. (1996) *Pressure Sore Prevention*. Whurr Publishers Ltd, London.

Stephens, M. (2001) *Guidelines for the Prevention and Treatment of Pressure Sores*. North Manchester Healthcare NHS Trust, Manchester.

Sutton, J. C. & Wallace, W. A. (1990) Pressure sores: the views and practices of senior hospital doctors. *Clinical Rehabilitation*, **4**, 137–43.

Torrance, C. (1983) *Pressure Sores: Aetiology, Treatment and Prevention*. Croom Helm, London.

Waterlow, J. (1988) Prevention is cheaper than cure. *Nursing Times*, **84** (25), 69–70.

Watkinson, G. (2002) Promoting Health. In: *Foundations of Nursing Practice: Making the Difference* (eds Hogston, R. & Simpson, P. M.), Palgrave Macmillan, Hampshire.

Wounds UK: www.wounds-uk.com

Young, J. B. & Dobrzanski, S. (1992) Pressure sores: epidemiology and current management concepts. *Drugs and Ageing*, **2** (1), 42–57.

Young, J. & Roper, T. A. (1996) The role of the doctor in the management of pressure sores. *Journal of Tissue Viability*, **7** (1), 18–23.

10 Continuing Professional Development

INTRODUCTION

As this is the final chapter of the book the author would like to conclude by discussing the importance of continuing professional development in your own practices and reminding you of some the dos and don'ts of pressure area care.

Pressure area care is a constantly changing area of practice. Manufacturing companies are continuously researching and developing new equipment for the prevention of pressure ulcers, with the wound care companies striving to develop a dressing that can treat pressure ulcers in an effective and efficient manner. Guidelines, protocols and policies, both at a national and local level, continue to be updated, as new evidence and research transpires regarding the prevention and treatment of pressure ulcers. This chapter will briefly discuss the importance of maintaining your own knowledge base and the sharing of knowledge with others.

LEARNING OBJECTIVES

By the end of this chapter the reader will be enabled to:

❑ Discuss the importance of continuing professional development
❑ Identify some areas of care that are not based upon evidence

The importance of continuing professional development has been a recurring theme throughout the chapters of this book. However, it cannot be stressed enough that all practitioners who are involved in pressure area care must undertake education and training to ensure that their knowledge base is up-to-date. Continuing professional development is not just about attending study days or undertaking formalised courses of study, but it also encompasses discussing relevant issues with specialists, reading relevant specialist journals and texts and reflecting upon the knowledge you have gained through undertaking these activities. All practitioners should adopt the concept of lifelong learning.

The Government, in line with its recommendations for clinical governance initiatives, has made it clear that healthcare areas must ensure that professional development plans (PDPs) are developed for clinical staff. These PDPs are developed in conjunction with the member of staff and their manager or senior clinical staff member and are designed to allow the two people to discuss their learning needs and the needs of the service. They provide a framework to plan how to meet the educational needs by developing competencies and accessing appropriate educational programmes to support learning. These plans can be developed for a one, two, or three year period, dependent upon local guidelines. They allow all practitioners to be able to develop their own educational needs and they help ensure that practice is updated and based on the best available evidence.

Education that promotes the use of evidence-based practice in pressure area care will not only benefit the patient but will help to prepare practitioners to deliver high standards of care. Sackett *et al.* (1997) identified that the move towards an all-graduate nursing profession had emphasised the need for research to become a fundamental aspect of nurse education and this has further enhanced the move towards evidence-based practice. This is definitely an issue that relates well to today's nurse education system by the fact that the moves towards an all-graduate profession are gaining pace, with the Royal College of Nursing supporting this as the way forward for nursing.

Engaging in your own professional development activities plays an important and vital role in ensuring that the importance of evidence-based practice is highlighted and that theory and practice are linked together to maintain a quality service. Remember that as a qualified practitioner you are responsible and accountable for your own actions. If you fail to exercise sufficient care, and in doing so you cause injury or harm to the patient, you will be considered negligent. When delivering safe and effective nursing care you are not only ensuring that your care is evidence based, but also that you are making informed decisions regarding the care to be delivered. McHale and Tingle (2003) state that a nurse could breach his or her legal duty of care by not keeping up-to-date with major new developments in their speciality. Therefore, nurses have a professional and legal duty to keep themselves updated with developments in nursing practice.

Maintaining registration

When you have qualified you will be offered a preceptorship period at your chosen workplace. This will normally last between three to six months and will give you the opportunity to consolidate the knowledge and skills you have learnt over your three-year training period. In addition to this, you will be required to re-register with the Nursing and Midwifery Council every three years. This entails providing details of your qualifications, area of work and evidence that you have maintained your professional knowledge and competence by completing a minimum of five days' study over the three years. Practitioners are also expected to maintain a professional portfolio; the Nursing and Midwifery Council may wish to see your profile that should detail your career progress, continuing education and your development plans. You can, therefore, see that continuing your professional development in all areas of your work, as well as pressure area care, is vitally important when you qualify. The Department of Health (1999) stated:

'We expect every nurse, midwife and health visitor to understand fully the obligations associated with professional regulation and accountability. . . . We expect them to maintain and improve their professional knowledge and competence at the very least to the minimum required during each registration cycle, and to acknowledge any limitations in knowledge and competence . . .'

Best practice

Student nurses visit many different areas during their training period and are often faced with a variety of techniques and ideas regarding pressure area care. There may be times when you witness some aspects of ritualised practice. In these cases it may be useful for you to question the rationale, evidence and/or research that supports this practice. If you are unsure as to whether or not the care is evidence based then you may wish to discuss it in more detail with your tissue viability specialist who will be able to offer you advice and guidance. You may also wish to read relevant texts and journals that will further enhance your knowledge base and understanding of the issues (refer to Appendix One).

Remember that you do not want to do any harm to your patient and if you are unsure as to whether or not you should be carrying out certain practices ask yourself: 'will these actions cause harm to my patient?'. If the answer is 'yes' to this then do not carry out the procedure, but do bear in mind that some procedures may cause some discomfort to the patient although they will still benefit them. For example, the administration of an intramuscular injection. You should also ask yourself: 'will my patient benefit as a result of this action?'. By asking yourself these questions you should be able to apply your knowledge and assess the potential benefit of performing this procedure to your patient.

Box 10.1 highlights some of the dos and don'ts of pressure area care. The examples presented are based on ritualistic practice and not on the best available evidence. If you should

---

Box 10.1 Dos and don'ts of pressure area care.

- Do ensure that an interdisciplinary approach is adopted for all aspects of pressure area care. This includes referring patients to the relevant professionals, e.g. specialist nurses, physiotherapists, occupational therapists, dieticians, etc.
- Do document all care administered, in a legible fashion. This will include choice of pressure redistributing equipment, choice of wound dressing and the rationale for that choice.
- Do ensure that all patient care is individualised and based on the best available evidence. Ritualised practice should be avoided.
- Do not rub or massage pressure areas as this causes friction and possible further damage to the deeper tissues.
- Do not rub or massage in barrier creams. Use them sparingly.
- Do use appropriate pressure redistributing equipment following individualised patient assessment.
- Do reposition patients that are being nursed on pressure-redistributing equipment as per their individualised care plan. This includes patients that are sitting in a chair. Ensure that the chair is the correct height for the patient and is not damaged.
- Do clean wounds when they are dirty.
- Do not clean wounds with gauze or cotton wool balls as they may shed fibres causing a focus for infection.
- Do not undertake any procedure if you have not been taught it and always seek advice from a competent practitioner if you are unsure as to how to perform a procedure.

---

witness them in practice the author advises you to ask the staff for the rationale for using them.

CONCLUSION

This chapter has highlighted the importance of maintaining your own professional development and has identified some areas of practice that are not based upon the evidence. Throughout your nursing career you will need to keep your knowledge base updated and ensure that the practice you deliver is based upon the best available evidence. Remember that as a qualified practitioner you will be required to re-register with the Nursing and Midwifery Council every three years and may be required to provide evidence of your learning. This may be demonstrated through the submission of your learning profile, so it is important that you do keep your knowledge and skills up-to-date throughout your career.

Good luck in your future careers!

SELF-ASSESSMENT
After reading this chapter you should now take some time to reassess your knowledge base.

Reflection

Take some time to reflect upon the knowledge you have gained and how you will implement it into your own practice.

What knowledge did I possess prior to reading this chapter?

What do I know now?

How will my practice change as a result of attaining this knowledge?

Do I need to discuss with anyone practices I have witnessed that are not evidence-based in relation to my new knowledge?

If so, who will I speak to?

REFERENCES

Department of Health (1999) *Making a Difference: Strengthening the Nursing, Midwifery and Health Visiting Contribution to Health and Healthcare.* Department of Health, London.

McHale, J. & Tingle, J. (2003) *Law and Nursing.* 2nd edn. Butterworth Heinmann, Edinburgh.

Sackett, D. L., Strans, S. E., Richardson, W. S., Rosenberg, W. & Haynes, R. B. (1997) *How to Teach Evidence-based Medicine: How to Practice and Teach EBM.* 1st edn. Churchill Livingstone, New York.

Glossary of Terms

Accountable	Responsible for something or to someone.
Acute wounds	Usually traumatic or surgical. They usually begin with a solitary, sudden insult and proceed to heal in an orderly manner without complication.
Angiogenesis	The growth of new blood vessels.
Antiseptics	A non-toxic disinfectant, which can be applied to skin and has the ability to destroy vegetative compounds, such as bacteria, by preventing their growth.
Bacteria	Any of the small unicellular micro-organisms of the class Schizomycetes.
Blanching hyperaemia	The distinct erythema caused by reactive hyperaemia, when the skin blanches or whitens if light finger pressure is applied, indicating that the patient's microcirculation is intact.
Capillary	One of the tiny blood vessels joining arterioles and venules.
Chronic wound	A wound with a prolonged inflammatory phase that may cause extended healing time.
Competent	Possessing the skills and abilities required for lawful, safe and effective professional practice without direct supervision.

Debridement	The removal of foreign material and devitalised tissue or contaminated tissue from the wound surgically, chemically or by autolysis.
DNA (deoxyribonucleic acid)	A large double stranded helical nucleic acid molecule, found principally in the chromosomes of the nucleus of the cell, that is the carrier of genetic information.
Devitalised tissue	Dead tissue.
Epitheliasation	One of the latter stages of wound healing. Completion of the epidermal covering by epithelial cells, normally pinkish in colour.
Erythema	A flushing of the skin due to the dilatation of the blood capillaries in the dermis.
Full thickness wounds	Destruction of epidermal and dermal layers. Loss of nerve endings, blood vessels, hair follicles and sweat glands. Deeper tissues such as muscle, bone or tendon may also be involved.
Granulation	Phase of healing without proliferation. The wound bed looks granular. Highly vascular due to the formation of new blood vessels, red in colour.
Growth factors	A subclass of cytokines, proteins that are used for cellular communication. Their particular role is to promote cell proliferation.
Incidence	Extent or frequency of occurrence, i.e. the number of people with a pressure ulcer over a given period of time.
Induration	The abnormal hardening of tissue.
Infection	An increase in the number of microorganisms, causing associated symptoms such as redness, swelling, oedema and heat.

Keratinocyte	A type of cell that makes up 95% of the cells of the epidermis. Keratinocytes migrate from the deeper layers of the epidermis and are finally shed from the surface of the skin.
Maturation	This is the final phase of healing, strengthening and reorganising collagen fibres.
Melanin	A dark brown to black pigment occurring in the hair, the skin and in the iris and choroid layer of the eyes.
Melanocytes	Cells within the epidermis of the skin that produce melanin.
Monocyte	A type of white blood cell with a kidney-shaped nucleus. It ingests bacteria and foreign debris.
Necrotic	Localised tissue death that occurs in groups of cells in response to disease or injury.
Neutrophil	A variety of granulocyte distinguished by the presence in its cytoplasm of fine granules that stain purple with Romanowsky stains. It is capable of killing and digesting bacteria and provides an important defence against infection.
Non-blanching hyperaemia	This is suggested where there is no skin colour change of the erythema when light finger pressure is applied, indicating a degree of micro-circulatory disruption, often associated with other clinical signs, such as, blistering, induration and oedema.
Oedema	The abnormal collection of fluid in interstitial spaces of tissues.
Parenteral	Administration of a substance by any other way than the mouth, e.g.

	introduction of a drug into the body by injection.
Phagocytosis	The engulfment and digestion of bacteria.
Prevalence	Widespread or common, i.e. the number of people with a pressure ulcer at a specific point in time, e.g. on one certain day.
Primary intention	Surgical wound or minor laceration where the skin edges are held together.
Proliferative phase	Infiltration of the wound site by new blood vessels and the growth and reproduction of the tissue as part of the healing process.
Pyrexia	A fever with a temperature of the body above 37°C.
Qualitative	Research that is mainly descriptive and involves collection and analysis of data concerned with meanings, attitudes and beliefs, rather than data that results in numerical counts that statistical inference can be drawn from. This type of research tends to generate masses of information that requires analysis and this in itself can be problematic as the data is often people's own opinions.
Quantitative	Research that is concerned with collecting and analysing data that focus on numbers and frequencies, seeking to establish cause and effect, rather than a meaning or experience.
Reactive hyperaemia	The characteristic bright flush of the skin associated with an increased volume of the pulse on the release of an obstruction to the circulation, or a vascular flush following the release of an occlusion of the

circulation, which is a direct response to incoming arterial blood.

Reasonable The case of Bolam v Friern Hospital Management Committee (1957, All ER 545) produced the following definition of what is reasonable. 'The test is the standard of the ordinary skilled man exercising and professing to have that special skill. A man need not posses the highest expert skill at the risk of being found negligent . . . it is sufficient if he exercises the skill of an ordinary man exercising that particular art.'

Sloughy A typical white/yellow colour. It is made up of dead cells that have accumulated in the exudate.

Stirling system A grading system that is broken down into four parts.

Strike through The passage of blood or serous exudate from the wound onto the outer surface of the dressing.

Superficial wounds Epidermal damage.

Surrey system A grading system broken down into four parts.

Synthesise To form or put together.

Systemic infection Infection pertaining to the whole of the body, rather than to a localised area.

Tensile strength The maximum pressure that can be applied to the wound without causing it to break apart.

Toxins A poison, usually one produced by, or occurring in, a plant or organism.

Trauma Potential for the accentuated risk of accidental tissue injury, such as burns, wounds or a fracture.

Type I diabetes	Also known as juvenile onset diabetes or insulin dependent diabetes mellitus (IDDM).
Type II diabetes	Also known as mature onset diabetes or non-insulin dependent diabetes mellitus.
Venule	A small vein.

Appendix 1

Searching the literature

When you are learning about a new subject or developing your knowledge base you will read many different texts and journal articles and utilise the Internet to find out what people have written about your chosen subject. This is known as searching and reviewing the literature. Please be careful, as not everything you read will be based solely upon the best available evidence or research findings. Some of the information you read may well be the writer's own personal viewpoint and they may have no evidence to substantiate their claims. The Internet is a useful medium to gain knowledge but again, remember, it is the World Wide Web and, therefore, it will contain practices from all over the world not just the UK. Although the information found may be interesting it may not follow the accepted policies, protocols and guidelines that are in place in the UK.

Why search the literature?

Nurses need to be aware of the research and evidence underpinning their own practices, and they need to know what has been written in their chosen subjects. Much has been written regarding pressure area care and you must understand the underpinning rationales for your own practices if you are to ensure that clinical practice is up-to-date and evidence based. The Department of Health has stressed the importance of clinical governance and clinical effectiveness initiatives to reflect the quality of practice that is administered to patients.

Clinical governance is a term that you may already be familiar with. It is an umbrella term that encompasses the areas of evidence-based practice, policy audit, evaluation, accountability and performance. It identifies the importance of:

- Involving patients
- The public
- Nurses
- Medical staff
- Professions allied to medicine
- Making decisions that will promote good and prevent poor quality
- Encouraging people to intervene in unacceptable practices
- Making practitioners accountable for the care they administer

All trusts and healthcare settings will now have clinical governance committees in place that will discuss areas of good practice and how to improve and further develop quality issues throughout the workplaces.

Clinical effectiveness is one area of clinical governance and is about doing the right thing at the right time. All practitioners should be able to demonstrate that their nursing interventions maintain and improve health within the available resources. To be able to achieve this nurses must understand why they are doing what they do and be able to explain the underpinning theory behind their intervention. It is no good saying 'I did it like that because we always do it like that'. It is, therefore, vitally important that you keep up-to-date with new ideas and developments in practice, and one way that this may be achieved is through reading and reviewing the literature. Other ways include attending study days, conferences, further study, and by discussing practices with specialists. Remember that following an educational event you should take time out to reflect on your new knowledge; this should be documented in your reflective diary.

How do you find the information you need?

There are various avenues you may wish to take to find the information you require. You may go to the library and find books that relate to your chosen area or you may browse through journals that contain articles related to the information you want. As mentioned earlier, the Internet contains a plethora of information and also has the electronic versions of journals. However, you may feel a little overwhelmed by the amount of information that is there for you to choose from. It is useful if you have keywords that you can enter into the search engine that will help to refine your searches. You should have no more than six keywords. It is worth remembering that terminology in nursing often changes, for example, pressure ulcers used to be referred to as pressure sores or bed sores; therefore, if you are attempting to retrieve articles from a few years ago for comparison purposes, you may have to change your keywords. There are a number of useful databases that you can access; examples of these can be seen below.

Examples of databases:

Medline: produced by the United States Library of Medicine and covers over 4000 journals. medline.cos.com

Cumulative Index to Nursing and Allied Health Literature (CINAHL): produced in the United States and indexes over 500 journals with records being updated annually. www.cinahl.com

RCN Internet site: produced by the Royal College of Nursing and is updated regularly. The site offers links to many other websites. www.rcn.org.uk

British Nursing Index: updated annually and offers over 9000 references. www.bni.org.uk

Cochrane Database: well-respected database offering reviews for a variety of subject areas. www.nelh.nhs.uk/cochrane.asp

Department of Health: this website allows you to view and download the Department of Health's papers. You can find the most recent publications here, plus access to past publications. www.dh.gov.uk

Nursing and Midwifery Council: this site allows you to access all the NMC's publications. www.nmc-uk.org

National Institute for Clinical Excellence (NICE): this site allows you to view the NICE guidelines for a variety of areas. www.nice.org.uk

Many of these sites only allow access through a subscription, but you should be able to access them through your local university library, providing you are a library member, and many of the trusts and healthcare areas subscribe to them. When you have collected the information you want, do not forget to make notes of the references, so if necessary you can find the information at a later date.

Review of the literature

Now you have the information you want, you need to review it. The introduction to each article should offer you an overview of the contents. Ask yourself: did the article refer to other important works in that area, or were there others that should have been considered? If the article you are reading is based upon numbers of participants, then how many are there in the group being researched, for example, if it is based on five people's views, then is this really a valid and reliable view to be considering?

Obviously, as a novice reading the literature it may be difficult for you to differentiate between a strong, well balanced piece of research or evidence, as opposed to a weak piece. However, it is useful to be aware that not everything you read will be exact. If in doubt consult a specialist in the area you are reading about and they will be able to offer advice and guide you.

As a student nurse, the best starting point will probably be one of your lecturers who has an interest in the area you wish to develop your knowledge in. They will be able to advise you as to who are the most respected writers and where to begin your searches. Do not forget that there are organisations such as the Tissue Viability Society, who will happily offer you advice.

Appendix 2

Clinical Guideline 7

Pressure Ulcer Prevention

Pressure Ulcer Risk Assessment and Prevention, Including the Use of Pressure-relieving Devices (Beds, Mattresses and Overlays) for the Prevention of Pressure Ulcers in Primary and Secondary Care*

* Incorporates the recommendations in *Inherited Clinical Guideline B* published by the Institute in April 2001

This guidance is written in the following context:
This guidance represents the view of the Institute, which was arrived at after careful consideration of the evidence available. Health professionals are expected to take it fully into account when exercising their clinical judgment. The guidance does not, however, override the individual responsibility of health professionals to make decisions appropriate to the circumstances of the individual patient, in consultation with the patient and/or guardian or carer.

CONTENTS

The following guidance is evidence based. The recommendations in this document are derived from two clinical guidelines, *Pressure Ulcer Risk Assessment and Prevention* and *Clinical Practice Guideline for Pressure-relieving Devices: the Use of Pressure-relieving Devices (Beds, Mattresses and Overlays) for the Prevention of Pressure Ulcers in Primary and Secondary Care* (see Section 5), which use different grading schemes. In the guideline on pressure ulcer risk assessment and prevention, evidence grading was 1, 2 and 3; in the guideline on pressure-relieving devices, recommendations were graded A, B, C and D. The grading schemes are described in Appendix 2A (p. 203). Summaries of the evidence on which the guidance is based are provided in the full guidelines (see Section 5).

The guideline on pressure ulcer risk assessment and prevention was published in 2001*. Its recommendations have been incorporated into this document, but the evidence used to develop it was not reviewed or updated during the development of the guideline on pressure-relieving devices.

1 GUIDANCE

The recommendations in this document are relevant to:

- those who are vulnerable to or at elevated risk of developing pressure ulcers
- families and carers
- healthcare professionals who share in caring for those who are vulnerable to or at elevated risk of developing pressure ulcers
- those with responsibility for purchasing pressure-relieving devices

---

* The recommendations were published by NICE in April 2001: National Institute for Clinical Excellence (2001) Pressure Ulcer Risk Management and prevention. *Inherited Clinical Guideline* B. National Institute for Clinical Excellence, London.

1.1 Risk assessment and prevention

1.1.1 Identifying individuals vulnerable to or at elevated risk of pressure ulcers

1.1.1.1 Assessing an individual's risk of developing pressure ulcers should involve both informal and formal assessment procedures. `3`

1.1.1.2 Risk assessment should be carried out by personnel who have undergone appropriate training to recognise the risk factors that contribute to the development of pressure ulcers and know how to initiate and maintain correct and suitable preventative measures. `3`

1.1.1.3 The timing of risk assessment should be based on each individual case. However, it should take place within six hours of the start of admission to the episode of care. `3`

1.1.1.4 If an individual is considered not to be vulnerable to or at elevated risk of pressure ulcers on initial assessment, reassessment should occur if there is a change in an individual's condition that increases risk (see Section 1.1.3). `3`

1.1.1.5 All formal assessments of risk should be documented/recorded and made accessible to all members of the interdisciplinary team. `3`

1.1.2 Use of risk assessment tools

1.1.2.1 Risk assessment tools should only be used as an aide-memoire and should not replace clinical judgement. `1`

1.1.3 Risk factors

1.1.3.1 An individual's potential to develop pressure ulcers may be influenced by the following intrinsic risk factors, which therefore should be considered when performing a risk assessment:

- reduced mobility or immobility
- sensory impairment
- acute illness
- level of consciousness
- extremes of age
- vascular disease
- severe chronic or terminal illness
- previous history of pressure damage
- malnutrition and dehydration

2

1.1.3.2 The following extrinsic risk factors are involved in tissue damage and should be removed or diminished to prevent injury: pressure, shearing and friction.

2

1.1.3.3 The potential of an individual to develop pressure ulcers may be exacerbated by the following factors, which therefore should be considered when performing a risk assessment: medication and moisture to the skin.

2

1.1.4 Skin inspection

1.1.4.1 Skin inspection should occur regularly and the frequency determined in response to changes in the individual's condition in relation to either deterioration or recovery.

3

1.1.4.2 Skin inspection should be based on an assessment of the most vulnerable areas of risk for each patient. These are typically: heels; sacrum; ischial tuberosities; parts of the body

3

affected by anti-embolic stockings; femoral
trochanters; parts of the body where pressure,
friction or shear is exerted in the course of an
individual's daily living activities; parts of the
body where there are external forces exerted by
equipment and/or clothing; elbows; temporal
region of skull; shoulders; back of head and toes. **3**

Other areas should be inspected as necessitated
by the patient's condition.

1.1.4.3 Individuals who are willing and able should be
encouraged, following education, to inspect their
own skin. **3**

1.1.4.4 Individuals who are wheelchair users should use
a mirror to inspect the areas that they cannot see
easily or get others to inspect them. **3**

1.1.4.5 Healthcare professionals should be aware of the
following signs, which may indicate incipient
pressure ulcer development: persistent erythema;
non-blanching hyperaemia, previously identified
as non-blanching erythema; blisters;
discolouration; localised heat; localised oedema
and localised induration. In those with darkly
pigmented skin: purplish/bluish localised areas
of skin; localised heat that, if tissue becomes
damaged, is replaced by coolness; localised
oedema and localised induration. **3**

1.1.4.6 Skin changes should be documented/recorded
immediately. **3**

1.2   Pressure ulcer prevention

1.2.1   Positioning

1.2.1.1   Individuals who are vulnerable to or at elevated
          risk of pressure ulcer development should be
          repositioned and the frequency of repositioning
          determined by the results of skin inspection and
          individual needs, not by a ritualistic schedule.
          3

1.2.1.2   Repositioning should take into consideration
          other relevant matters, including the patient's
          medical condition, their comfort, the overall
          plan of care and the support surface.
          3

1.2.1.3   Positioning of patients should ensure that:
          prolonged pressure on bony prominences is
          minimised, bony prominences are kept from
          direct contact with one another, and friction
          and shear damage is minimised.
          3

1.2.1.4   A repositioning schedule, agreed with the
          individual, should be recorded and established
          for each person vulnerable to pressure ulcers.
          3

1.2.1.5   Individuals or carers, who are willing and able,
          should be taught how to redistribute weight.
          3

1.2.1.6   Manual handling devices should be used
          correctly in order to minimise shear and friction
          damage. After manoeuvring, slings, sleeves or
          other parts of the handling equipment should
          not be left underneath individuals.
          3

1.2.2   Seating

1.2.2.1   Seating assessments for aids and equipment
          (otherwise known as assistive technologies)
          should be carried out by trained assessors who
          3

have the acquired specific knowledge and expertise (for example, physiotherapists or occupational therapists). | 3

1.2.2.2 Advice from trained assessors with acquired specific knowledge and expertise should be sought about correct seating positions. | 3

1.2.2.3 Positioning of individuals who spend substantial periods of time in a chair or wheelchair should take into account distribution of weight, postural alignment and support of feet. | 3

1.2.2.4 The management of a patient in a sitting position is important. Even with appropriate pressure relief, it may be necessary to restrict sitting time to less than two hours until the condition of an individual with an elevated risk changes. | D

1.2.2.5 No seat cushion has been shown to perform better than another, so this guideline makes no recommendation about which type to use for pressure redistribution purposes. | 3

1.2.3 Use of aids

1.2.3.1 The following should not be used as pressure-relieving aids: water-filled gloves; synthetic sheepskins*; doughnut-type devices. | 3

1.2.4 Pressure-relieving devices (beds, mattresses and overlays)

1.2.4.1 Decisions about which pressure-relieving device to use should be based on cost considerations | D

* Since the guideline on pressure ulcer prevention and assessment was published (see Section 5) a study in Australia has suggested that natural sheepskin may be effective in pressure ulcer prevention.

and an overall assessment of the individual. **D**
Holistic assessment should include all of the
following:

- identified levels of risk
- skin assessment
- comfort
- general health state
- lifestyle and abilities
- critical care needs
- acceptability of the proposed pressure-
  relieving equipment to the patient and/or
  carer

and should not be based solely on scores from risk
assessment tools.

1.2.4.2 All individuals assessed as being vulnerable to **B**
pressure ulcers should, as a minimum provision,
be placed on a high-specification foam mattress
with pressure-relieving properties.

1.2.4.3 Although there is no research evidence that high- **D**
tech pressure-relieving mattresses and overlays
are more effective than high-specification
(low-tech) foam mattresses and overlays,
professional consensus recommends that
consideration should be given to the use of
alternating pressure or other high-tech
pressure-relieving systems:

- as a first-line preventative strategy for people
  at elevated risk as identified by holistic
  assessment
- when the individual's previous history of
  pressure ulcer prevention and/or clinical
  condition indicates that he or she is best
  cared for on a high-tech device
- when a low-tech device has failed

1.2.4.4 All individuals undergoing surgery and assessed D
as being vulnerable to pressure ulcers should, as
a minimum provision, be placed on either a
high-specification foam theatre mattress or other
pressure-redistributing surface.

1.2.4.5 The provision of pressure-relieving devices D
needs a 24-hour approach. It should include
consideration of all surfaces used by the
patient.

1.2.4.6 Support surface and positioning needs should be D
assessed and reviewed regularly and determined
by the results of skin inspection, and patient
comfort, ability and general state. Thus,
repositioning should occur when individuals
are on pressure-relieving devices.

1.2.4.7 A pressure ulcer reduction strategy should D
incorporate a coordinated approach to the
acquisition, allocation and management of
pressure-relieving equipment. The time elapsing
between assessment and use of the device
should be specified in this strategy.

1.2.5 Education and training

1.2.5.1 All healthcare professionals should receive 2
relevant training or education in pressure
ulcer risk assessment and prevention.

1.2.5.2 An interdisciplinary approach to the training 3
and education of healthcare professionals
should be adopted.

1.2.5.3 Training and education programmes for 3
healthcare professionals should include:

- risk factors for pressure ulcer development 3
- pathophysiology of pressure ulcer development
- the limitations and potential applications of risk assessment tools
- skin assessment
- skin care
- selection of pressure-relieving equipment
- use of pressure-relieving equipment
- maintenance of pressure-relieving equipment
- methods of documenting risk assessments and prevention activities
- positioning to minimise pressure
- shear and friction damage including the correct use of manual handling devices
- roles and responsibilities of interdisciplinary team members in pressure ulcer management
- policies and procedures regarding transferring individuals between care settings
- providing education and information to patients

1.2.5.4 Healthcare professionals with recognised training 3 in pressure ulcer management should cascade their knowledge and skills to their local healthcare teams.

1.2.5.5 Individuals vulnerable to or at elevated risk of 3 developing pressure ulcers who are able and willing should be informed and educated about risk assessment and resulting prevention strategies. This strategy should, where appropriate, include carers.

1.2.5.6 Education for individuals vulnerable to pressure D ulcers, and their carers, should include providing information verbally and in writing on the following:

- the risk factors associated with developing pressure ulcers   **D**
- the sites that are of the greatest risk of pressure damage
- how to inspect skin and recognise skin changes
- how to care for skin
- methods for pressure relief/reduction
- the use and maintenance of pressure-relieving devices
- where patients/carers can seek further advice and assistance
- the need for immediate visits to a healthcare professional if signs of damage are noticed

Equipment safety

Equipment safty is an important issue in relation to the use of pressure-relieving devices. In particular, cross infection is possible where equipment is inadequately decontaminated between patients (Orr *et al.* 1994*) and injury is possible if users of such equipment (patients, carers and health professionals) have not been educated about appropriate use. Guideline users are therefore referred to the standards on medical devices management and decontamination of reusable medical devices (Medical Devices Agency, 2002a,b†). Users of these guidelines are encouraged to familiarise themselves with the sections of these documents relevant to the use and decontamination of pressure-relieving devices. Anecdotal evidence suggests that if there is no access to adequate decontamination facilities it may be desirable to lease pressure-relieving devices. The advantage of leasing in these circumstances is that the devices can be returned to the manufacturer for thorough decontamination after each patient use.

* Orr, K.E., Gould, F.K., Perry, J.S. *et al.* (1994) Therapeutic beds: the Trojan horses of the 1990s? *Lancet*, 344; 65–66.

†Medical Devices Agency (2002a). *Medical Devices Management.* Medical Devices Agency, London.

Medical Devices Agency (2002b). *Decontamination of Reusable Medical Devices.* Medical Devices Agency, London.

2   NOTES ON THE GUIDANCE

2.1   Terminology used in the guidance on pressure-relieving devices

- Where the term 'carer' is used, this refers to unpaid carers as opposed to paid carers (for example, careworkers).

- There is much debate in the literature and amongst experts about the appropriateness of the term 'pressure-relieving'. For the purposes of this guidance, 'pressure-relieving' is used as an umbrella term for all pressure-reducing and pressure redistributing devices.

- Pressure ulcers have also been known previously as pressure sores, bed sores and decubitus ulcers.

- The terms 'vulnerable to pressure ulcers' and 'at elevated risk of pressure ulcers' are used in this guideline rather than the terms 'at risk' and 'at very high risk'. The latter terms imply that there are reliable cut-off points for identifying risk, yet there is little evidence to show that using a pressure ulcer risk assessment tool is better than clinical judgement for assessing risk, or that allocation of pressure-relieving devices can be linked to risk assessment tools.

- Pressure-relieving devices (from Cullum *et al.*, 2001*)

    Low-tech devices: these provide a conforming support surface that distributes the body weight over a large area. They include the following:

* Cullum, N., Nelson, E. A., & Sheldon, T. (2001) Systematic reviews of wound care management (5): pressure-relieving beds, mattresses and cushions for the prevention and treatment of pressure sores. In: Cullum, N., Nelson, E. A., Flemming, K. *et al.* Systematic reviews of wound care management: (5) beds; (6) compression; (7) laser therapy, therapeutic ultrasound, electrotherapy and electromagnetic therapy. *Health Technology Assessment*, **5** (9).

Standard foam mattress

Alternative foam mattresses/overlays (for example, high-specification foam, convoluted foam, cubed foam); these are conformable and aim to redistribute pressure over a larger contact area

Gel-filled mattresses/overlays

Fluid-filled mattresses/overlays

Fibre-filled mattresses/overlays

Air-filled mattresses/overlays

High-tech devices: these are dynamic systems that include the following:

Alternating-pressure mattresses/overlays: the patient lies on air-filled sacs, which sequentially inflate and deflate and relieve pressure at different anatomical sites for short periods; these devices may incorporate a pressure sensor

Air-fluidised beds/mattresses/overlays: warmed air is circulated through fine ceramic beads covered by a permeable sheet; these allow support over a larger contact area

Low-air-loss overlays/mattresses/beds: the patient is supported on air-filled sacs inflated at a constant pressure, through which air is able to pass

Turning beds/frames (kinetic beds): beds that either aid manual repositioning of the patient or reposition the patient by motor-driven turning and tilting

2.2   Scope of the guidance

Pressure ulcers have a profound negative effect on the physical, social and financial realms of people's lives and are also distressing for their carers. Although the guideline does not cover treatment of existing pressure ulcers, its recommendations will be useful in preventing pressure ulcers on other areas of the patient's body and further pressure damage to existing pressure ulcers.

The recommendations in this document are derived from two sources: the guideline on pressure ulcer risk assessment and prevention, published by NICE in 2001, and the guideline on pressure-relieving devices, commissioned by NICE (see Section 5).

2.2.1   Pressure ulcer risk assessment and prevention

This section of the guideline was commissioned by the Department of Health from the RCN (Royal College of Nursing) before NICE was established. It followed closely the development brief that was agreed at the time of commissioning, and was originally published by NICE in 2001 as a stand-alone document.

The aim of the guideline on pressure ulcer risk assessment and prevention was to reduce the occurrence of pressure ulcers by giving healthcare professionals guidance on the early identification of patients vulnerable to developing pressure ulcers, the provision of preventative interventions, and by identifying practice that may be harmful or ineffective.

2.2.2   Pressure-relieving devices

The guideline on the use of pressure-relieving devices (specifically beds, mattresses and overlays) for the prevention of pressure ulcers for use in the NHS in England and Wales was commissioned to supplement the NICE guideline on pressure ulcer risk assessment and prevention. The scope of the guidance on the use of pressure relieving devices was established at the start of the development of this guideline, following a period of consultation; it is available from www.nice.org.uk/article.asp?a=29296. It was subsequently decided to combine the new guideline with the recommendations in the 2001 guideline to produce this document.

The recommendations on pressure-relieving devices apply to patients of all ages, but in developing the guideline no trials were identified that applied specifically to children.

The main area examined by this section of the guideline was:

- the most clinically effective and cost-effective beds, mattresses or overlays for preventing pressure ulcers

Additional areas included:

- the evidence for linking risk assessment to the allocation of pressure-relieving devices
- differences in comfort and acceptability ratings, ease of use, and adverse events between the different devices
- whether quality of life varies with use of different pressure-relieving devices
- the groups at particularly high risk of developing pressure ulcers
- the costs of preventing pressure ulcers, including the costs of pressure relieving devices for both the health services and patients vulnerable to pressure ulcers and their carers

The guideline presents recommendations for good practice based on the best available evidence of clinical and cost effectiveness. However, there was a lack of formal economic evaluations and quality-of-life data, and the clinical effectiveness data were of variable quality. Furthermore, very little published research relating to paediatric care exists. Consequently, not all areas examined could be fully addressed. Evidence published after October 2002 was not considered.

2.3   Principles of practice

The following principles are important in relation to these guidelines. These principles are based on those published by the Royal College of Nursing (RCN, 2001*).

* Royal College of Nursing (2001) *Pressure Ulcer Risk Assessment and Prevention*. Royal College of Nursing, London. Available from www.rcn.org.uk and www.nice.org.uk/Docref.Asp?d=16423

2.3.1   Person-centred care

- Patients and their carers should be made aware of the guideline and its recommendations and be referred to the version for the public.
- Patients and their carers should be involved in shared decision-making about pressure-relieving devices.
- Health professionals are advised to respect and incorporate the knowledge and experience of people who have been at long-term risk of developing pressure ulcers and have been self-managing this risk.
- Patients and their carers should be informed about their risk of developing pressure ulcers, especially when they are transferred between care settings or discharged home.

2.3.2   A collaborative interdisciplinary approach to care

- All members of the interdisciplinary team should be aware of the guidelines, and all care should be documented in the patient's healthcare records.

2.3.3   Organisational issues

- An integrated approach to pressure ulcer prevention is needed, with a clear strategy and policy supported by management.
- Care should be delivered in a context of continuous quality improvement, where improvements to care following guideline implementation are the subject of regular feedback and audit.
- Commitment to and availability of education and training are needed to ensure that all staff, regardless of profession, are given the opportunity to update their knowledge base and are able to implement the guideline recommendations.
- Patients should be cared for by personnel who have undergone appropriate training in recognising the risk factors that

of data on patient comfort as well as physiological measures, would be of value.

- Further research evaluating the effect of educational programmes is needed. Limited research suggests that educational programmes may have an effect in reducing pressure ulcer incidence. Clinicians' reported experiences indicate that education is key to effective pressure area management. However, more conclusive research evidence is needed on what should be included in training, at what level, how training and education should be delivered, and how competency is assessed and updated.

- There is also a paucity of research exploring the perceptions and experiences of individuals vulnerable to pressure ulcers (and their carers), their involvement in pressure area care and their educational requirements. This information might be uncovered by well-designed studies using a mixture of qualitative and quantitative approaches to data collection through, for example, semi-structured interviews and focus groups, and pre-validated quality of life measures.

Pressure-relieving devices

- Comparisons are needed, in groups at elevated risk, of alternating pressure devices with:

  lower tech alternatives (for example, different types of high-specification foam mattresses and other constant low-pressure devices)
  other high-tech devices (for example low-air-loss and air-fluidised devices)

  Comparisons should include the cost and cost effectiveness of devices, as well as the difference in relative risk of using the devices, for different groups of individuals.

- Investigation is needed of the impact of pressure ulcers on the quality of life of individuals and carers, and of the

199

quality of life achieved with different forms of pressure relief.

- Evaluation of the impact and effectiveness of formal assessment at the point of entry into healthcare (including acute care, care homes and in the community) and the impact of delays to this process would be valuable.

- The need for and frequency of manual repositioning should be investigated, including:

  requirement for repositioning on any pressure-relieving device

  methods of repositioning individuals on different pressure-relieving devices

  nursing time involved in repositioning

- Large-scale prospective epidemiological studies are needed to improve understanding of risk factors and the relative contribution they make to the development of pressure ulcers, and to facilitate the development of risk assessment tools based on adequate prospective research.

5   FULL GUIDELINES

The recommendations in this document are derived from two guidelines.

The guideline on pressure ulcer risk assessment and prevention was a part of the Institute's inherited clinical guidelines work programme. It was commissioned by the Department of Health before the Institute was established in April 1999. The developers worked with the Institute to ensure, in the time available, that the guideline was subjected to validation and to consultation with stakeholders. However, it was not possible to subject it to the full guideline development process that the Institute has now adopted. The full guideline – *Pressure Ulcer Risk Assessment and Prevention*, which was produced by the Royal College of Nursing (RCN) – is available on the

NICE website (www.nice.org.uk/Docref.asp?d=16423). The recommendations from the guideline were published by NICE in April 2001 (*Inherited Clinical Guideline* B).

The National Institute for Clinical Excellence commissioned the development of the guidance on pressure-relieving devices from the National Collaborating Centre for Nursing and Supportive Care. The Centre established a Guideline Development Group, which reviewed the evidence and developed the recommendations. The full guideline, *Clinical Practice Guideline for Pressure-relieving Devices: the Use of Pressure-relieving Devices (Beds, Mattresses and Overlays) for the Prevention of Pressure Ulcers in Primary and Secondary Care*, is published by the National Collaborating Centre for Nursing and Supportive Care; it is available on the NICE website (www.nice.org.uk) and on the website of the National Electronic Library for Health (www.nelh.nhs.uk).

The members of the Guideline Development Groups are listed in Appendix B. Information about the Guideline Advisory Committee and the independent Guideline Review Panel is given in Appendix C.

The booklet *The Guideline Development Process – Information for the Public and the NHS* has more information about the Institute's guideline development process. It is available from the Institute's website and copies can also be ordered by telephoning 0870 1555 455 (quote reference N0038).

6   RELATED NICE GUIDANCE

Woundcare suite

This document is part of a suite of clinical guidelines on woundcare management, including the prevention of skin breakdown. Other guidelines in the suite include:

- Infection control: prevention of healthcare-associated infection in primary and community care. Published June 2003. See www.nice.org.uk/cat.asp?c=71774
- Management of pressure ulcers – guideline under development, planned for publication in May 2005. For further details, see www.nice.org.uk/cat.asp?c=33925
- Management of patients with venous leg ulcers – guideline developed by the Royal College of Nursing (see www.rcn.org.uk/resources/guidelines.php) and being updated by the RCN at the time this NICE guideline was issued
- The management of surgical wounds – guideline under development, planned for publication April 2006. For further details, see www.nice.org.uk/cat.asp?c=33930
- General principles of the management of wounds – guideline under development.

7   REVIEW DATE

The process of reviewing the evidence is expected to begin four years after the date of issue of this guideline. Reviewing may begin earlier than four years if significant evidence that affects the guideline recommendations is identified sooner. The updated guideline will be available within two years of the start of the review process.

Versions of this document written for people vulnerable to pressure ulcers, their families and carers, and the public are available from the NICE website (www.nice.org.uk) and from the NHS Response Line (telephone 0870 1555 455 and quote reference number N0331 for a version in English only and reference number N0332 for a version in English and Welsh).

APPENDIX 2A: GRADING SCHEME

The grading scheme used in *Pressure Ulcer Risk Assessment and Prevention* (see Section 5) was adapted from Waddell, G., Feder, G., McIntosh, A. *et al.* (1996) *Low Back Pain Evidence Review*. Royal College of General Practitioners, London. Grading was as follows.

Evidence

(1) Generally consistent finding in a majority of multiple acceptable studies.
(2) Either based on a single acceptable study, or a weak or inconsistent finding in multiple acceptable studies.
(3) Limited scientific evidence that does not meet all the criteria of acceptable studies or absence of directly applicable studies of good quality. This includes expert opinion.

'Acceptable' for this guideline refers to those that have been subjected and approved by a process of critical appraisal. For further details see: Rycroft-Malone, J. & McInnes, E. (2001) *Pressure Ulcer Risk Assessment and Prevention Guideline: Technical Report*. Royal College of Nursing, London. Available from www.rcn.org.uk

The grading scheme and hierarchy of evidence used in *Clinical Practice Guideline for Pressure-relieving Devices: the Use of Pressure-relieving Devices (Beds, Mattresses and Overlays) for the Prevention of Pressure Ulcers in Primary and Secondary Care* (see table), is from Eccles and Mason (2001).

Recommendation grade	Evidence
A	Directly based on category I evidence
B	Directly based on:
	• category II evidence, **or**
	• extrapolated recommendation from category I evidence
C	Directly based on:
	• category III evidence, **or**
	• extrapolated recommendation from category I or II evidence
D	Directly based on:
	• category IV evidence, **or**
	• extrapolated recommendation from category I, II or III evidence

Evidence category	Source
I	Evidence from:
	• meta-analysis of randomised controlled trials, **or**
	• at least one randomised controlled trial
II	Evidence from:
	• at least one controlled study without randomisation, **or**
	• at least one other type of quasi-experimental study
III	Evidence from non-experimental descriptive studies, such as comparative studies, correlation studies and case–control studies
IV	Evidence from expert committee reports or opinions and/or clinical experience of respected authorities

Adapted from Eccles, M. & Mason, J. (2001) How to develop cost-conscious guidelines. *Health Technology Assessment*, **5** (16).

APPENDIX 2B: THE GUIDELINE DEVELOPMENT GROUPS

Pressure ulcer risk assessment and prevention

Guideline Developers
Ms Jo Rycroft-Malone
Project Officer (RCN Institute)

Ms Elizabeth McInnes
Formerly Project Officer RCN Institute

Expert Consensus Group
Ms Maureen Benbow
Tissue Viability Nurse, Leighton Hospital

Dr Mary R. Bliss
Consultant Geriatrician, Bryning Day Hospital

Dr Michael Clark
Senior Research Fellow, University of Wales College of Medicine, Cardiff

Ms Linda Clarke
Patient Services Manager, Spinal Injuries Association, London

Mrs Carol Dealey
Research Fellow, University Hospital Birmingham NHS Trust

Dr Krzysztof Gebhardt
Clinical Nurse Specialist for Pressure Sore Prevention, St George's Hospital, London

Ms Deborah Hofman
Clinical Nurse Specialist, Wound Healing Unit, The Churchill Hospital, Oxford

Ms Pennie Roberts
Head of Physiotherapy Studies, Leeds Metropolitan University

Dr Shyam Rithalia
Senior Lecturer, University of Salford

Professor John Young
Consultant Geriatrician St Lukes Hospital, Bradford

Pressure-relieving devices
Dr Paul Yerrell (group leader)
Oxford Brookes University

Mr Malcolm Blanch
Carers UK

Dr Michael Clark
Wound Healing Research Unit,
University of Wales College of Medicine

Mr Mark Collier
United Lincolnshire Hospitals NHS Trust

Mr Louis Hecht
Tissue Viability Society

Mr Nick Malone
Oxford Radcliffe Trust

Dr Jed Rowe
Royal College of Physicians

Dr Eileen Scott
North Tees & Hartlepool NHS Trust

Mrs Fiona Stephens
Royal College of Nursing (now East Kent PCTs)

Mr Adam Thomas
RADAR

Dr Elizabeth White
College of Occupational Therapists

National Collaborating Centre for Nursing and Supportive Care
Ms Sue Boyt
Administrator

Dr Gill Harvey
Director

Ms Rosa Legood
Health Economist
(seconded from Health Economics Research Centre, University of Oxford)

Ms Elizabeth McInnes
Senior R&D Fellow

Mr Robin Snowball
Information Scientist
(seconded from Cairns Library, John Radcliffe Hospital, Oxford)

Mr Edward Weir
Centre Manager

APPENDIX 2C: THE GUIDELINES ADVISORY COMMITTEE AND GUIDELINE REVIEW PANEL

Guidelines advisory committee

At the time the guideline on risk assessment and prevention of pressure ulcers was published, the Guidelines Advisory Committee (GAC) was a standing committee of the Institute. It had responsibility for agreeing the scope and commissioning brief for clinical guidelines and for monitoring progress and methodological soundness. The GAC considered responses from stakeholders and advised the Institute on the acceptability of the guidelines it had commissioned. It has since been superseded by the Guideline Review Panel. Details of the membership of the GAC are shown in the NICE guideline on pressure ulcer risk assessment and prevention (see Section 5).

Guideline review panel

The Guideline Review Panel is an independent panel that oversees the development of the guideline and takes responsibility for monitoring its quality. The Panel includes experts on guideline methodology, health professionals and people with experience of the issues affecting patients and carers. The members of the Guideline Review Panel for the guideline on pressure-relieving devices were as follows.

Mrs Judy Mead
Head of Clinical Effectiveness, Chartered Society of Physiotherapy

Dr Marcia Kelson
Director, Patient Involvement Unit for NICE

Mrs Joyce Cormie
Patient representative

Mrs Gill Hek
Principal Lecturer, University of West of England

Mrs Karen Cowley
Practice Development Nurse, York Hospital

Mrs Jill Freer
Head of Clinical Governance and Quality Development, Leicestershire, Northamptonshire and Rutland Strategic Health Authority

Miss Amanda Wilde
Reimbursements and Outcomes Manager, Convatec Ltd

APPENDIX 2D: TECHNICAL DETAIL ON THE CRITERIA
FOR AUDIT OF THE USE OF PRESSURE-RELIEVING
DEVICES FOR THE PREVENTION OF PRESSURE ULCERS
IN PRIMARY AND SECONDARY CARE

The audit criteria below are to assist with implementation of
the guideline recommendations. The criteria presented here
are considered to be the key criteria associated with the guideline recommendations. They are suitable for use in primary
and secondary care, for all individuals vulnerable to or at elevated risk of developing pressure ulcers who are admitted to
hospital for medical or surgical management or who are discharged to an extended care facility or home.

- Users of these guidelines are reminded that the criteria
  presented here should be used in conjunction with the
  audit criteria presented in *Pressure Ulcer Risk Assessment and
  Prevention* (RCN, 2001*).
- Equipment allocation cannot be driven by risk assessment
  alone, and percentages of individuals within different risk
  groups who should be allocated specific equipment cannot
  be specified.
- As well as formal risk assessment, clinical judgement, patient condition, lifestyle and prior experiences of
  pressure-relieving devices require consideration when allocating devices.

Possible objectives for an audit

Audits can be carried out in different care settings to ensure
that individuals who are vulnerable to developing pressure
ulcers, or who are at elevated risk of developing pressure
ulcers, are offered appropriate pressure-relieving devices, are

---

* Royal College of Nursing (2001) *Pressure Ulcer Risk Assessment and
Prevention*. Royal College of Nursing, London. Available from
www.rcn.org.uk and www.nice.org.uk/Docref.asp?d=16423

involved in decisions about their care, and have been informed about the rationale and use of pressure-relieving devices.

Because the allocation of pressure-relieving devices is only one part of a pressure ulcer reduction strategy, pressure ulcer incidence is not an appropriate subject for audit to evaluate the implementation of this guideline.

People that could be included in an audit

An audit could be conducted in settings where people are at elevated risk of developing pressure ulcers – for example, intensive care unit, orthopaedic, neurological, and spinal injuries units and selected patients discharged to the community.

Data sources and documentation of audit

Systems for recording the necessary information (which will provide data sources for audit) should be agreed by trusts.

Whatever method is used for documentation, the process and results of risk assessment and equipment allocation should be accessible to all members of the multidisciplinary team. In relation to risk assessment, this should include name of the risk assessment tool used, evidence of scores and evidence of holistic assessment prior to allocating pressure-relieving devices.

The factors taken into consideration when choosing the most appropriate pressure-relieving device for a patient, the devices allocated, and the reasons for any changes in devices should be documented.

The fact that patients vulnerable to pressure ulcers, and their carers, have been informed about pressure ulcer prevention using pressure-relieving devices and educated about the use, operation and management of the equipment should be documented. Patients vulnerable to pressure ulcers and carers should be directly questioned about their satisfaction with, and the adequacy of, the information provided and this should be documented in the patient notes or in another source as agreed by the trust.

Trusts should establish a system to record when staff have been educated in pressure ulcer risk assessment and the handling of pressure-relieving devices and should implement a process to review education needs relating to risk assessment and pressure-relieving devices.

Measures that could be used as a basis for an audit

The table overleaf suggests measures that could be used as a basis for audit.

Criterion	Standard	Exception	Definition of terms
Allocation of pressure-relieving devices (includes mattresses and overlays, both high-tech and low-tech) • **Recommendations 1.2.4.1–1.2.4.4, 1.2.4.7**			
(1) Pressure-relieving devices are offered to individuals vulnerable to, or at elevated risk of developing, pressure ulcers as determined by holistic assessment (the results of which are documented in the patient's healthcare notes), within an agreed time-scale.	100%	The device is not appropriate for the individual (for example a high-tech device that may be unstable for patients with fractures). The patient declines a particular device.	The holistic assessment as described in recommendation 1.2.4.1 will assist with the identification of patients deemed vulnerable to, or at elevated risk of developing, pressure ulcers.
(2) Individuals cared for on pressure-relieving devices are moved to an alternative device within an agreed timescale if their condition changes.	100%	The device has been reported by the patient or their carer, or is known to the health professional to be harmful or unacceptable to that individual.	
Repositioning while being cared for on pressure-relieving devices • **Recommendations 1.2.2.4, 1.2.4.5, 1.2.4.6**			

Criterion	Standard	Exception	Definition of terms
(1) Individuals cared for on a pressure-relieving device have their repositioning needs and sitting times determined by a regular review of individual needs.	100%	None.	
Patient/carer information			
• **Recommendation 1.2.5.6**			
(1) Individuals who are allocated pressure-relieving devices, and their carers, receive written and verbal information about the device, its operation and management and its role in the prevention of pressure ulcers. This information includes the lay version of this guideline (see section 7).	100%	None.	Trusts should agree on the type of information to be made available, when, and by whom.
Staff education/knowledge			
• **Recommendation 1.2.5.3**			
(1) Staff caring for people vulnerable to or at elevated risk of pressure ulcers are educated in: • risk assessment • the safe use and operation of pressure-relieving devices • the monitoring of any adverse consequences associated with pressure-relieving devices	100%	None.	Trusts should ensure that each clinical setting has access to advice on handling pressure-relieving devices (including safety, decontamination and the reporting of adverse events).

Calculation of compliance

Compliance (%) with each measure described in the table above is calculated as follows.

$$\frac{\text{Number of patients whose care is consistent with the } \textbf{criterion } \textit{plus} \text{ number of patients who meet any } \textbf{exception} \text{ listed}}{\text{Number of patients to whom the } \textbf{measure} \text{ applies}} \times 100$$

Clinicians should review the findings of measurement, identify whether practice can be improved, agree on a plan to achieve any desired improvement and repeat the measurement of actual practice to confirm that the desired improvement is being achieved.

APPENDIX 2E: GLOSSARY

Partially based on *Clinical Epidemiology Glossary* by the Evidence-Based Medicine Working Group, www.ed. ualberta.ca/ebm, *Information for National Collaborating Centres and Guideline Development Groups* (NICE, 2001)*, Guidelines on Pressure Ulcer Risk Assessment and Prevention (NICE, 2001; RCN, 2001)* and Cullum *et al.* (2001) *Health Technology Assessment*, **15** (9).

Air-fluidised beds/mattresses/overlays: warmed air is circulated through fine ceramic beads covered by a permeable sheet; these allow support over a larger contact area.

Alternating-pressure mattresses/overlays: the patient lies on air-filled sacs, which sequentially inflate and deflate and relieve pressure at different anatomical sites for short periods; these devices may incorporate a pressure sensor.

Basic 'old-style' hospital mattresses: usually a single piece of polyurethane foam confined by a non-stretch plastic or nylon cover which has few pressure-relieving properties.

Case–control study: a study in which the effects of a treatment or management approach in a group of patients are compared with the effects of a similar group of people who do not have the clinical condition (the latter is called the control group).

Clinical effectiveness: the extent to which an intervention (for example, a device or treatment) produces health benefits (that is, more good than harm).

Cost effectiveness: the cost of an intervention per unit of benefit. In cost-effectiveness analysis, the outcomes of different interventions are converted into health gains for which a cost can be associated – for example, cost per additional pressure ulcer prevented.

*Available from www.nice.org.uk

Economic evaluation: comparative analysis of alternative courses of action in terms of both their costs and consequences.

Effectiveness: the extent to which interventions achieve health improvements in real practice settings.

Epidemiological study: a study that looks at how a disease or clinical condition is distributed across geographical areas.

Erythema: non-specific redness of the skin which can be localised or general in nature and which may be associated with cellulitis, infection, prolonged pressure or reactive hyperaemia.

Fibre-filled overlays/mattresses: synthetic fibres in a series of connected cushions. The fibre may be silicone coated, or formed into balls to reduce shear and friction.

Fluid-filled overlays or mattresses: the fluid conforms to the micro-contours of the body, consistently moving and reducing shear as well as providing overall pressure relief.

Gel (viscoelastic) filled pads: frequently used on operating theatre tables to protect head, heels and ankles.

Health technology assessment: the process by which evidence on the clinical effectiveness and the costs and benefits of using a technology in clinical practice is systematically evaluated.

High-specification foam pressure-relieving devices ('foam alternatives'): for example, high-specification foam, convoluted foam, cubed foam; these are conformable and aim to redistribute pressure over a large contact area.

High-tech devices: an alternating support surface where inflatable cells alternately inflate and deflate.

Hyperaemia

Reactive hyperaemia: the characteristic bright flush of the skin associated with an increased volume of the pulse on the release of an obstruction to the circulation, or a vascular flush following the release of an occlusion of the circulation which is a direct response to incoming arterial blood.

Blanching hyperaemia: the distinct erythema caused by reactive hyperaemia, when the skin blanches or whitens if light finger pressure is applied, indicating that the patient's microcirculation is intact.

Non-blanching hyperaemia (previously identified as non-blanching erythema): indicated when there is no skin colour change of the erythema when light finger pressure is applied, indicating a degree of microcirculatory disruption often associated with other clinical signs, such as blistering, induration and oedema.

Induration: the abnormal hardening of tissue (or organ).

Low-air-loss overlays/mattresses/beds: the patient is supported on air-filled sacs inflated at a constant pressure, through which air is able to pass.

Low-tech devices: a conforming support surface that distributes the body weight over a large area.

Meta-analysis: a statistical method of summarising the results from a group of similar studies.

Oedema: increase in fluid in intercellular space, swelling.

Overlay: term used to describe surfaces placed on top of a standard mattress or operating table.

Pressure-relieving: equipment that removes pressure from different areas of the body.

Randomised controlled trial (RCT): a clinical trial in which the treatments are randomly assigned to participants. The random allocation eliminates bias in the assignment of treatment to individuals and establishes the basis for the statistical analysis.

Systematic review: a way of finding, assessing and using evidence from studies (usually RCTs) to obtain a reliable overview.

Turning beds/frames (kinetic beds): beds that either aid manual repositioning of the individual or reposition the patient by motor-driven turning and tilting.

Appendix 3
Pressure Ulcers*

DEFINITION

Pressure ulcer (sometimes referred to as pressure sore/bed sore/decubitus ulcer) = identified damage to an individual's skin due to the effects of pressure together with, or independently from, a number of other factors, e.g. shearing, friction, moisture, etc. Reproduced by kind permission of HMSO, London.

Agreed patient/client focused outcome	
The condition of the patient's/client's skin will be maintained or improved	
Indicators/information that highlights concerns which may trigger the need for benchmarking activity:	
Audits-documentation/care pathways/ guidance Pressure ulcer – incidence & prevalence figures Product usage/availability Patient satisfaction surveys, complaints, figures and analysis Educational audits/student placement feedback	Litigation/clinical negligence scheme for trusts Professional concern Media reports Commission for Health Improvement reports

	FACTOR	BENCHMARK OF BEST PRACTICE
(1)	Screening/assessment	**For all** patients/clients identified as **'at risk'**, screening **progresses to further assessment**

*For guidance on how to use this Appendix see pp. xv–xix.

(2)	Who undertakes the assessment	Patients/clients are assessed by **assessors** who have the required **specific knowledge and expertise**, and have **ongoing updating**
(3)	Informing patients/ clients/carers (prevention and treatment)	Patients/clients and carers have ongoing **access to information** and have the **opportunity to discuss** this and its relevance to their individual needs, with a registered practitioner
(4)	Individualised plan for prevention and treatment of pressure ulcers	**Individualised** documented **plan** agreed with multidisciplinary team **in partnership** with patient/client/ carers, with **evidence of ongoing reassessment**
(5)	Pressure ulcer prevention – repositioning	The patient's/client's need for repositioning has been assessed/ documented/met/evaluated with evidence of **ongoing reassessment**
(6)	Pressure ulcer prevention – redistributing support surfaces	Patients at risk of developing pressure ulcers **are cared for on** pressure redistributing support surfaces that meet their individual needs, including comfort
(7)	Pressure ulcer prevention – availability of resources – equipment	Patients/clients have **all the equipment they require** to meet their individual needs
(8)	Implementation of individualised plan	The plan is **fully implemented in partnership** with the multidisciplinary team/patients/clients/carers
(9)	Evaluation of interventions by a registered practitioner	An evaluation which incorporates patients/clients/carers **participation in forward planning**, is documented

Key sources

Department of Health. NHS Executive. (1994) Pressure sores: a preventable problem. *VFM Update*, 12.

Risk Assessment and Prevention of Pressure Ulcers: a Clinical Practice Guideline [in press].

University of Leeds. Nuffield Institute for Health, University of York. NHS Centre for Reviews and Dissemination. (1995) The prevention and treatment of pressure sores. *Effective Health Care*, **2**, 1.

FACTOR 1   SCREENING/ASSESSMENT

Patients/ clients pressure ulcers or their risk of developing a pressure ulcer is not **ascertained**.	Patients/clients are **not consistently screened** for the presence of or risk of developing pressure ulcers.	Patients/clients are screened but this does not lead to **more detailed assessment** of those patients/ clients identified as 'at risk'.	For all patients/clients identified as 'at risk' screening **progresses to further assessment**
E	**D**	**C** **B**	**A**

Note: screening should always be undertaken at initial contact and the need for reassessment of patients/clients should be continuously considered.

Screening: a process of identifying patients who already have or who are at risk of developing a pressure ulcer. It requires sufficient knowledge for clinical judgement. Those at high level of risk require referral for a further comprehensive assessment.

Assessment: a formal, comprehensive and systematic process in which a range of specific methods/tools can be used to identify and quantify the patient's/client's risk.

At risk: individuals who have, as a result of screening, been identified as having or as being vulnerable to the development of pressure ulcers.

Evidence which comparison group members agree would justify best practice (A)

Possibly to include: (1) Policies, procedures and guidelines (2) Staffing and workforce (3) Education, training & development (4) Information/communication (5) Resources: facilities & equipment (6) Specificity to patient/client needs (include ethnic/cultural/age related/special needs) (7) Partnership working with clients, carers, multidisciplinary teams, social care, etc.

Evidence: *(to be completed by comparison group members for like to like comparison)*

Statements to stimulate comparison group discussion around best practice

State how patients/clients are assessed as being 'at risk'

State the components of the screening assessment

State who completes the screening assessment and how this is recorded

State when the screening assessment is undertaken

State who completes the full assessment

State what is included in full assessment and assessment tools used

State if a manual handling assessment is included

State the evidence base for assessment and how this is updated to reflect current evidence

FACTOR 2   WHO UNDERTAKES THE ASSESSMENT

Patients/ clients are assessed by **assessors who do not have the required specific knowledge and expertise**.	Some patients/clients are assessed by assessors who have **some training**.	Patients/clients are assessed by **assessors who have the required specific knowledge and expertise**.	Patients/ clients are assessed by assessors who have the required specific knowledge and expertise and have **ongoing updating**.
E	**D**	**C** **B**	**A**

Unqualified staff, students/patients/carers can screen patients if they have received the necessary education and training and have been assessed as competent to undertake the screening, but accountability remains with the registered practitioner. Registered practitioners who have received the necessary education and training and have been assessed as competent to undertake the assessment.

Evidence which comparison group members agree would justify best practice (A)

Possibly to include: (1) Policies, procedures and guidelines (2) Staffing and workforce (3) Education, training & development (4) Information/communication (5) Resources: facilities & equipment (6) Specificity to patient/client needs (include ethnic/cultural/age related/special needs) (7) Partnership working with clients, carers, multidisciplinary teams, social care, etc.

Evidence: *(to be completed by comparison group members for like to like comparison)*

Statements to stimulate comparison group discussion around best practice

State how knowledge and expertise is acquired (for screening and assessment)

State the way in which knowledge, skills and attitudes are updated on an ongoing basis

State the mechanisms for assessing competence of the screeners and assessors

Describe how specialist assessment is accessed if required

State how assessment is documented and accessed by caring team

FACTOR 3   INFORMING PATIENTS/CLIENTS AND CARERS (PREVENTION AND TREATMENT)

E	D	C	B	A
Patients/clients and carers have **no access to information**.	Patients/clients and carers have **access to relevant information but no opportunity to discuss** with a registered practitioner.	Patients/clients and carers have access to information and have had the opportunity to **discuss this and its relevance to their individual needs** with a registered practitioner.	Patients/clients and carers have **ongoing access** to information and have the opportunity to discuss this and its relevance to their individual needs with a registered practitioner.

Registered practitioner has the specific knowledge base to lead an informed discussion with the patient/client/carer.

Evidence which comparison group members agree would justify best practice (A)

Possibly to include: (1) Policies, procedures and guidelines (2) Staffing and workforce (3) Education, training & development (4) Information/communication (5) Resources: facilities & equipment (6) Specificity to patient/client needs (include ethnic/cultural/age related/special needs) (7) Partnership working with clients, carers, multidisciplinary teams, social care, etc.

Evidence: *(to be completed by comparison group members for like to like comparison)*

Statements to stimulate comparison group discussion around best practice

State the range and format available to meet patient/client/carer individual needs including religious/cultural/linguistic, age-related and special needs (language/tapes/videos/leaflets)

State the evidence base for the information

State how patient's understanding of information is verified and choices documented

State how the sharing and understanding of information is recorded

State the ongoing training and education received by registered practitioners to enable them to access, share, explain and explore information (including orientation and during supervision and PDP)

FACTOR 4   INDIVIDUALISED PLAN FOR PREVENTION AND TREATMENT OF PRESSURE ULCERS

No plan or no documented plan.	Documented plan **not** **individualised** based on patient/client assessment.	Documented plan is **individualised** but does not include agreement from multidisciplinar y team in partnership with patient/client/ carers.	Individualised documented plan agreed with multidisciplinar y team **in** **partnership** with patient/client/ carers.	**Individualised** documented **plan** agreed with multidisciplinar y team **in** **partnership** with patient/client/ carers, **with** **evidence of** **ongoing** **reassessment**.
E	**D**	**C**	**B**	**A**

Plan – centred on correction or minimisation of intrinsic and extrinsic factors.

Evidence which comparison group members agree would justify best practice (A)

Possibly to include: (1) Policies, procedures and guidelines (2) Staffing and workforce (3) Education, training & development (4) Information/communication (5) Resources: facilities & equipment (6) Specificity to patient/client needs (include ethnic/cultural/age related/special needs) (7) Partnership working with clients, carers, multidisciplinary teams, social care, etc.

Evidence: *(to be completed by comparison group members for like to like comparison)*

| |
| |
| |
| |
| |

Statements to stimulate comparison group discussion around best practice

Describe how responsibilities (of patients/clients/carers/multidisciplinary team members) with regard to treatments, interventions, milestones and targets are negotiated and agreed (including removal of barriers to effective communication, e.g. linguistic, age-related and special needs).

State the evidence that all plans are underpinned by best evidence

State the mechanisms in place to ensure review of plans and evaluation

FACTOR 5 PRESSURE ULCER
PREVENTION – REPOSITIONING

The patient's/client's **need for repositioning has not been assessed**.	The patient's/client's need for repositioning has been assessed and documented but **not met**.	The patient's/client's need for repositioning has been assessed/documented **and met**.	The patient's/client's need for repositioning has been assessed/documented/met and **evaluated**.	The patient's/client's need for repositioning has been assessed/documented/met/evaluated with evidence of **ongoing reassessment**.
E	D	C	B	A

Note: repositioning applies to patients/clients being cared for on any type of surface.

Equipment should be used effectively to avoid any damage to the patient/client/carer as a result of repositioning.

Evidence which comparison group members agree would justify best practice (A)

Possibly to include: (1) Policies, procedures and guidelines (2) Staffing and workforce (3) Education, training & development (4) Information/communication (5) Resources: facilities & equipment (6) Specificity to patient/client needs (include ethnic/cultural/age related/special needs) (7) Partnership working with clients, carers, multidisciplinary teams, social care, etc.

Evidence: *(to be completed by comparison group members for like to like comparison)*

Statements to stimulate comparison group discussion around best practice

State equipment available to enable correct moving and handling and positioning, including pillows, etc.

State training and education programmes in place

State patient/carer information available for repositioning

State policies/guidelines in use re: health and safety, manual handling, equipment use, etc.

FACTOR 6 PRESSURE ULCER PREVENTION – REDISTRIBUTING SUPPORT SURFACES

Patients/clients at risk of developing pressure ulcers **are not given the opportunity** of being placed on pressure redistributing support surfaces.	Patients at risk of developing pressure ulcers **have the opportunity** to be placed on pressure redistributing support surfaces.	Patients at risk of developing pressure ulcers **are cared for on** pressure redistributing support surfaces that meet their individual needs (including comfort).
E	**D** **C** **B**	**A**

Pressure redistributing/reducing support surfaces: static and active pieces of equipment, i.e. mattresses, cushions that assist in spreading the patient's body weight in order to minimise the effects of pressure.

At risk patients: individuals who have been identified as vulnerable to the development of pressure ulcers as a result of initial screening/full assessment and informed clinical judgement (see Factor 1).

Evidence which comparison group members agree would justify best practice (A)

Possibly to include: (1) Policies, procedures and guidelines (2) Staffing and workforce (3) Education, training & development (4) Information/communication (5) Resources: facilities & equipment (6) Specificity to patient/client needs (include ethnic/cultural/age related/special needs) (7) Partnership working with clients, carers, multidisciplinary teams, social care, etc.

Evidence: *(to be completed by comparison group members for like to like comparison)*

Statements to stimulate comparison group discussion around best practice

State what redistributing support surfaces are used: state records kept
State arrangements for surface cleanliness and maintenance and replacement
State the infection control policies in place and their relevance to surface cleaning
State how person's comfort is assessed and assured
State the process for ordering, delivery and monitoring of support surfaces
State the patient information available including consideration of information to meet religious/cultural and special needs

FACTOR 7   PRESSURE ULCER PREVENTION –
AVAILABILITY OF RESOURCES – EQUIPMENT

Patients/clients are **not provided** with any pressure ulcer prevention equipment.	Patients/clients **are provided** with equipment but it is **not the equipment required to meet their individual needs**.	Patients/clients are provided with a **limited range** of the equipment required to meet their individual needs.	Patients/clients have **the equipment they require** to meet their individual needs.
E	D	C	B A

Equipment: e.g. pressure redistributing equipment including; seating/mattresses/specialist beds/bed frames/electric profiling bed frames/moving and handling/hoists/footwear/insoles.

Types of dressing evidenced as a preventative measures are included.

Evidence which comparison group members agree would justify best practice (A)

Possibly to include: (1) Policies, procedures and guidelines (2) Staffing and workforce (3) Education, training & development (4) Information/communication (5) Resources: facilities & equipment (6) Specificity to patient/client needs (include ethnic/cultural/age related/special needs) (7) Partnership working with clients, carers, multidisciplinary teams, social care, etc.

Evidence: *(to be completed by comparison group members for like to like comparison)*

Statements to stimulate comparison group discussion around best practice

State the range of equipment available

State the barriers that limit access to or use of equipment

State policies in place for use of equipment

State arrangements for equipment cleanliness, repair, maintenance and replacement

State the infection control policies in place and their relevance to equipment cleaning

State the process for ordering, delivery and monitoring of equipment

State how patients/clients are made aware of the equipment available and how to use it safely

FACTOR 8   IMPLEMENTATION OF INDIVIDUALISED PLAN

No care given or not given **according to plan**.	**Some elements** of care are given according to plan.	The plan is **implemented but not in partnership** with the multidisciplinary team and patient/client/carers.	The plan is **fully implemented in partnership** with the multidisciplinary team/patients/ clients/ carers.
E	**D**	**C** **B**	**A**

Note: the inability to implement the plan leads to reassessment.

Evidence which comparison group members agree would justify best practice (A)

Possibly to include: (1) Policies, procedures and guidelines (2) Staffing and workforce (3) Education, training & development (4) Information/communication (5) Resources: facilities & equipment (6) Specificity to patient/client needs (include ethnic/cultural/age related/special needs) (7) Partnership working with clients, carers, multidisciplinary teams, social care, etc.

Evidence: *(to be completed by comparison group members for like to like comparison)*

Statements to stimulate comparison group discussion around best practice

State barriers to the implementation of planned care and how variance is recorded

State how multidisciplinary team is involved and involvement is documented

State how patients/clients are involved

State how carers are involved

State evidence of patient/carer training

State how religious/cultural/linguistic and special needs are addressed

FACTOR 9   EVALUATION OF INTERVENTIONS BY A REGISTERED PRACTITIONER

No evaluation of intervention s takes place.	Evaluation takes place but **not documented**.	**Evaluation is documented** but there is **no forward planning**.	An evaluation which includes **forward planning but patient/ client/carer views are not taken into account.**	An evaluation which **incorporates patient's/ client's/ carer's participation** in forward planning, is documented.
E	D	C	B	A

Note: the non-registered practitioner/patient/carer can state care delivered and report on progress made but is not expected to evaluate the effectiveness of intervention.

Evidence which comparison group members agree would justify best practice (A)

Possibly to include: (1) Policies, procedures and guidelines (2) Staffing and workforce (3) Education, training & development (4) Information/communication (5) Resources: facilities & equipment (6) Specificity to patient/client needs (include ethnic/cultural/age related/special needs) (7) Partnership working with clients, carers, multidisciplinary teams, social care, etc.

Evidence: *(to be completed by comparison group members for like to like comparison)*

| |
| |
| |
| |
| |
| |

Statements to stimulate comparison group discussion around best practice

State how patient/clients/carers are involved/participate

State how documentation reflects accurate and timely evaluation e.g. audit of records

State guidelines and policies in use that support forward planning

ACTION PLANNED TO DEVELOP PRACTICE
PRESSURE ULCERS

COMPILED BY: [_____] __/__/__

FOR: (Self/Team/Trust/Region) [_____]

AIM: PATIENT FOCUSED BEST PRACTICE =			Related factors
ACTION REQUIRED	**By whom**	**Date to complete**	**REFLECTION**

AIM: PATIENT FOCUSED BEST PRACTICE =			Related factors
ACTION REQUIRED	**By whom**	**Date to complete**	**REFLECTION**

AIM: PATIENT FOCUSED BEST PRACTICE =			Related factors
ACTION REQUIRED	**By whom**	**Date to complete**	**REFLECTION**

AIM: PATIENT FOCUSED BEST PRACTICE =			Related factors
ACTION REQUIRED	**By whom**	**Date to complete**	**REFLECTION**

AIM: PATIENT FOCUSED BEST PRACTICE =			Related factors
ACTION REQUIRED	**By whom**	**Date to complete**	**REFLECTION**

COMPARISON GROUP COLLATED SCORES
PRESSURE ULCERS

Comparison group: – (self/team/ practice/ward/area/directorate/trust)	Date scored: __/__/__	Date of comparison group meeting: __/__/__

(1) A = For all patients/clients identified as 'at risk' screening progresses to further assessment

Score Order A–E	Member (name/code)	Why score chosen/how justified?

(2) A = Patients/clients are assessed by assessors who have the required specific knowledge and expertise, and have ongoing updating

Score Order A–E	Member (name/code)	Why score chosen/how justified?

(3) A = Patients/clients and carers have ongoing access to information and have the opportunity to discuss this and its relevance to their individual needs, with a registered practitioner

Score Order A–E	Member (name/code)	Why score chosen/how justified?

(4) A = Individualised documented plan agreed with multidisciplinary team in partnership with patient/client/carers, with evidence of ongoing reassessment

Score Order A–E	Member (name/code)	Why score chosen/how justified?

(5) A = The patient's/client's need for repositioning has been assessed/documented/met/evaluated with evidence of ongoing reassessment

Score Order A–E	Member (name/code)	Why score chosen/how justified?

(6) A = Patients at risk of developing pressure ulcers are cared for on pressure redistributing support surfaces that meet their individual needs (including comfort)

Score Order A–E	Member (name/code)	Why score chosen/how justified?

(7) A = Patients/clients have the equipment they require to meet their individual needs

Score Order A–E	Member (name/code)	Why score chosen/how justified?

(8) A = The plan is fully implemented in partnership with the multidisciplinary team/patients/clients/carers

Score Order A–E	Member (name/code)	Why score chosen/how justified?

(9) A = An evaluation which incorporates patient's/client's/carer's participation in forward planning, is documented

Score Order A–E	Member (name/code)	Why score chosen/how justified?

SCORING SHEET
PRESSURE ULCERS

Score relates to practice by/on/in: (self/team/practice/ward/area/directorate/trust)			
Comparison group lead member:		**Date to be scored:** __/__/__ **By:** _____ (insert name)	**Date form to be returned:** __/__/__
Scored by:	**Date scored:** __/__/__	**Copied: Y/N**	**Posted on:** __/__/__
Date comparison group meeting to share good practice and compile action plan: __/__/__ **To be attended by:**_____(insert name)		**Re-score date agreed:** __/__/__	

SCORE:	**(1) Screening/assessment**	
	Why score chosen/how justified?	
SCORE:	**(2) Who undertakes the assessment?**	
	Why score chosen/how justified?	

SCORE:	**(3) Informing patients/clients/carers (prevention and treatment)** Why score chosen/how justified?
SCORE:	**(4) Individualised plan for prevention and treatment of pressure ulcers** Why score chosen/how justified?

SCORE:	(5) Pressure ulcer prevention – repositioning
	Why score chosen/how justified?

SCORE:	(6) Pressure ulcer prevention – redistributing support surfaces
	Why score chosen/how justified?

SCORE:	(7) Pressure ulcer prevention – availability of resources – equipment
	Why score chosen/how justified?

SCORE:	**(8) Implementation of individualised plan** Why score chosen/how justified?
SCORE:	**(9) Evaluation of interventions by a registered practitioner** Why score chosen/how justified?

Index